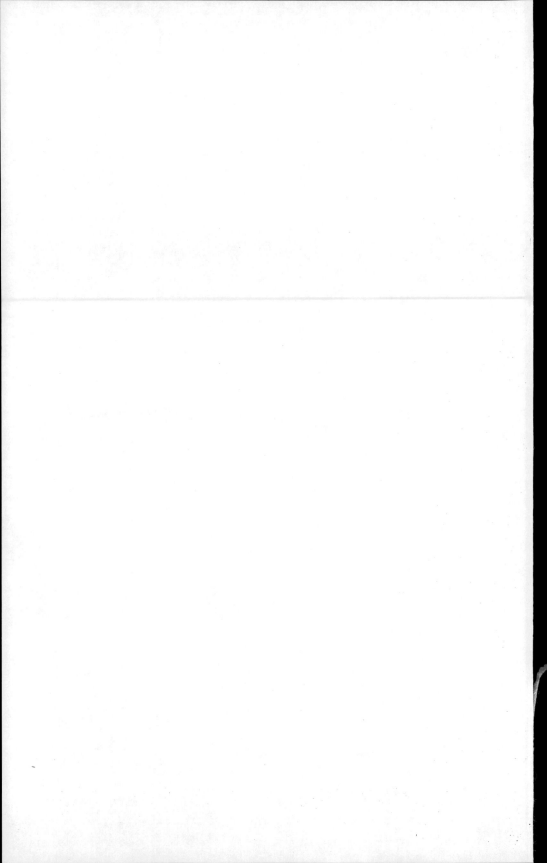

WOMEN: FIT AT FIFTY
A Guide for Living Long

Colleen,
    Keep up with all that inspires
you. Your story is one that others will enjoy.
Look towards that next 5k!

                                    Mary Macklin

Mary Kathryn Macklin, MSN, Cardiac Nurse Practitioner

authorHOUSE®

AuthorHouse™
1663 Liberty Drive
Bloomington, IN 47403
www.authorhouse.com
Phone: 1-800-839-8640

First published by AuthorHouse   10/24/2011

ISBN: 978-1-4670-4043-3 (sc)
ISBN:978-1-4670-4042-6 (hc)
ISBN: 978-1-4670-4041-9 (e)

Library of Congress Control Number: 2011917115

Printed in the United States of America

Any people depicted in stock imagery provided by Thinkstock are models, and such images are being used for illustrative purposes only. Certain stock imagery © Thinkstock.

This book is printed on acid-free paper.

The journey of a thousand miles begins with one step.
Lao Tzu

When I stand before God at the end of life, I would hope
that I would not have a single bit of talent left
and I could stay "I used everything you gave me"
Erma Bombeck

Dedicated to

My Mother, Mary Lagasse,
for showing me that
fitness is a way of life.

&

Dearest Margie,
taken from us far too young
despite doing all the right things.

Your friends are never gone
If you look to the sky
And pray.
(brandi carlile)

HOW TO USE THIS BOOK

Women: Fit at Fifty is written in the hopes of inspiring you, the reader, to evaluate your life style and make changes where necessary. The primary intent is to motivate you to start moving and to keep moving, no matter what type of movement you choose. There are chapters intended to teach you about certain physiologic processes which are directly affected by the behavioral choices you make and the diseases that result when less healthy choices are made. Other chapters offer suggestions and strategies to motivate you and help you to achieve your health goals. Lastly, the chapters relating stories about real women are included to show that we all face barriers, struggles and real life excuses that prevent us from doing things we know will be helpful.

The layout of the book is such that chapters build on each other. You can read the book from cover to cover. However, each chapter can stand alone if you choose to skip around. There are specific points repeated in a few chapters for those who do not read in order. Some chapters may need to be reread when you are lacking inspiration to stick with it. There are people who will read about all the women first, then go back and read other chapters as they see fit. If you are one of those, there are little vignettes within some of the chapters too so you can continue to be inspired by real people.

The appendices at the end are working tools to assist as you transition towards your goals. Each of these tools is discussed within the appropriate chapter but is repeated at the end so you can tear them out and keep handy when you need to review why you are doing such hard work to stay healthy. Several web sites are listed to provide additional resources for those who want to know more.

Finally, you can jump on to my Facebook page to get additional information, motivational tips and to talk to other women just like you who are looking towards a healthier way forward. Search Women: Fit at Fifty. On the site there are two videos available for demonstration purposes. One is a short set of arm exercises using light weights that can be done at home. The other is a series of abdominal exercises which are described in the "five minute rule". Feel free to email me at womenfitatfifty@gmail. com. I would love to hear from you.

DISCLAIMER

There are women who have underlying heart disease and do not yet have signs or symptoms. If you have not been exercising, you might be at risk of a problem. Before launching into an exercise program, it would be important to talk with your primary care provider to obtain their input and advice. Depending on your risk profile, a stress test may be recommended. If you do not have a stress test before hand and develop any symptoms when you start an exercise routine, take a break and contact your provider to discuss this further. Once you get the green light, go forward and enjoy.

ACKNOWLEDGEMENTS

This project has been a long term, time consuming task; often keeping me from being outside doing all the things I love. Many times, I have questioned the value of this book and whether I should continue or give it up. Often I have neglected the house work and other chores that demanded time and attention. Yet, each day at work I would encounter at least one woman who inspired me to continue. Some were fifty something year old women who either needed to, wanted to or already were doing the right thing. Others were older women like those described in the last chapter who reminded me why I needed to continue writing. Some were the younger women still with a chance to take charge and live long. The women who allowed me to write their stories also provided an incentive to keep going. All of you told me how important this work was and that I needed to finish. To all of you women, thank you for keeping me focused and motivated.

To my friends and colleagues who provide inspiration; Michele, Holly, Susan, LuAnn, Mike, Jan, Linda, Beth, Mark, Jason, Hilda, Jim, the yoga women, all of you at the Racquet Club and so many more; thank you. The Reach The Beach runners; Shelly, Marilyn, Amanda, Brent, Ralph, Charlene, Jen, Mike, Larry, Paul, Susan for giving me a reason to run and to write. You did not even know that your spirit spurred me on so many times when I wanted to give up. So keep going and training for those fun events. Thank you to anyone I have unintentionally neglected to name. I am sorry if I left you out.

My friends Mary, Kae and Mark helped me so much by reading sections and giving me honest input. Kae, thanks also for constantly checking in on my progress. I always wanted to tell you that I was making headway so you motivated me to push forward. Thanks to Mark and Michele for telling me I HAD to publish this no matter what, just when I needed the final inspiration. Thanks to my brother Fred for staying in shape and giving me the idea to write a second book about fifty year old men. Also thanks to my Dad and Pam for being so happy and believing in me.

My heartfelt thanks to my sister Jeanne, who always keeps going and staying strong, no matter what life delivers. And to my other sister, Karen, for all the advice and input and for telling me that "quitting is not an option". You have no idea how much that helped. Thanks to my mother for getting me going at a young age and for always telling me I look good even when I don't.

Lastly, my unending love and appreciation to my husband and children, Mike, Lauren, Ross and Grady and to Dekker, the dog. We have walked, hiked, skied and biked many miles together. We have seen many beautiful vistas and have many more ahead. Without you I would not be who I am and I would not have the joy in my life that I feel every day. I love you all so much.

FORWARD

It started the day after the short course triathlon. My husband, Mike, my friend, Susan and I were mountain bike riding at Bear Brook State Park in Pembroke, NH, me at the rear as usual. I was reflecting on the event, still high from from the adrenalin and the feeling of accomplishment. Susan had inspired and pushed me during training for the one third mile swim, 15 mile bike and 3 mile run. She had helped ease my anxiety by accompanying me for a course run-though two weeks earlier. My thoughts were already on next year and where I could speed up to improve on my time.

As I rode and thought, my mind kept going back to the feeling that I should have done better. At the end of the event, I was not terribly tired or worn out. Athletes often say that if they feel good when crossing the finish line, they have not really worked as hard as possible. That was definitely me. I liked to ease along and although pushed a bit, stretching to the limit was not really my style. I vacillated between feeling great and feeling disappointed with my results. Prior to the occasion, I had set a personal time goal to complete all three events and I had crossed the finish line in under my goal. Still I could not shake the feeling that I should have been faster. Finally, the realization came that I should be proud of what I had done, that I should not be downplaying the feat. I was fifty four years old and just crossing the finish line in a respectable time was a pretty good achievement.

As I reflected on the other people who competed, one woman in particular stuck in my mind. She was a rather heavy woman who I had passed on the early part of the bike ride. I saw her again as I was heading to the transition zone between the bike and run segments of the event.

She still had not reached the half-way point of the 15-mile bike course and was pushing her bike up the hill. All I could think was that she had a long way to go and the day was getting pretty warm. Later when I was leaving, there she was again just nearing the finish line of the bike portion. A car was trailing her with a big sign that said "Last Biker". I was one of the slower competitors and had already completed the event, relaxed, eaten, packed my stuff to leave and she still had to finish the run portion of the triathlon! Most of the other race competitors were done with only a small number still on the race course. My heart went out to her until I realized that this was commitment in the absolute. My admiration for this woman triathlete soared. I wished there was a marching band to spur her on and was very glad that many volunteers and fans still enthusiastically lined the running course and the finish line.

My mind wandered further to the variety of women in their fifties who had come out to participate in this fun happening. It was surprising that although some were quite athletic, there were equally as many women taking on a very significant challenge. There they were, women of all shapes and sizes waiting anxiously for the starting gun to fire. Some were accompanied by friends, some with daughters or sons, some with husbands, many with other women, probably even some who were alone, all prepared to take on the course ahead. All these women should be congratulated on what they were able to do.

I started thinking of the contrast of the women I had seen at the triathlon with many of those I care for in my daily work as a Cardiac Nurse Practitioner. As part of my work I conduct cardiac exercise stress tests. It astounds me each day, how out of shape, overweight, and at-risk so many people are. Many women my age and younger can't walk more than six minutes on a treadmill at less than 2.5 miles an hour. That actually is a very slow pace given that a moderately brisk walker can complete 4 miles in an hour. We are talking about people who cannot complete even six minutes. Often times, women (as well as men) have their stress test done for the indication of "shortness of breath with activities". Clearly there are some who truly have a cardiac problem and our job in the stress lab is to complete a diagnostic evaluation to help discover what their health issue might be. But when I look at many others, I already have a sense of why they are short of breath. Many are simply inactive and therefore deconditioned. Many are overweight and don't understand that it is the extra 20, 30, 40.... pounds that are causing their shortness of breath. Many of these people are so sedentary that a limited amount of exercise is beyond their capability. Many have never been educated or counseled about the health risks of high blood pressure, high blood sugar, heart disease, sedentary life style, excessive weight and smoking.

I also thought of how many women I know who have given up their activities and put on extra pounds as they aged. Many of my coworkers had grown in clothing size as the years went by and the pounds piled on. It is tragic to think about where these women will be in another ten years. How then to spread the word about simple steps that can be taken to either stay on or get back on the road to health. Alas, the book Women: Fit at Fifty was born.

This book is written for all the women out there who know they should do more to stay healthy. It is for women who want to change their behaviors but need a boost to get started. This is for women who have never exercised and think it is too late to start. It is for those of you who have strayed from an exercise routine and want to get back. And this is for women who have stayed active and need the support to continue. This book is also for those of you who have just been told that you need to change your life style to save your health. Women: Fit at Fifty is for all of you nearing or in your fifties who want to live a much longer, healthier life. It is for all the younger women who one day will be fifty. It is for women who have family and friends who love them. The time to start is now.

CONTENTS

Chapter 1

EXCUSES and PROCRASTINATION

By the time we reach our fifties, it is easy to feel that we are past the point where it matters if we stay active and fit. It may seem that the important years have passed by. The thought of beginning an exercise routine for a person who has never been particularly active or for someone who has let their activities slide, may be daunting. Habits are extremely well ingrained. Friendships and other relationships, especially marriages, are set in routines that may not include physical activities. Many people begin to think that it just does not matter any more because of how "old" they are. However, at the age of fifty there are so many years left to live and staying active will help to maintain a productive and healthy life through these years.

There is extensive research that has indisputably shown that exercise at any age, but especially as we get older, is essential to ward off disease, delay age related decline and to live longer. We know that the human body undergoes predictable physiological changes as we age. Some of these are obvious, like wrinkles developing on our faces and breasts which begin to sag while some are less obvious such as decreased elasticity of blood vessels and decline in lung function. As discussed in detail in the next chapter, it is well documented that routine physical activity can minimize some of the internal changes that occur and at least in part, prevent the development of chronic diseases. Daily exercise can also increase energy levels which tend to decline as we get older and improve ones outlook as we enter the "middle age" and "elderly" phases of our lives.

In regards to fitness, there are three main types of women. First, there are those who have adopted healthy life style behaviors to include a controlled diet and regular exercise. If you are in that group and are reading this book, it may be because you desire to learn more or to reinforce the benefits of your commitment. The second group includes those who do not habitually practice these behaviors. People in this group may not be interested or motivated to change their habits for any number of reasons. Those of you in this group who are reading this book may be curious yet not ready to believe these changes are worthwhile. Hopefully, after a few chapters you will become a believer.

The third group is those in the middle. This group generally includes women who want to change or know they should but they have not quite figured out how to get started. Perhaps you want to begin an exercise routine and just need the push to start. Perhaps you are exercising a little and now need the impetus to help you stick with it. Maybe you want to incorporate diet control strategies as you increase your exercise regime. Some of you may have recently been diagnosed with a condition that can be controlled with life style changes. If you are in this third group, keep reading. The strategies in these chapters will help you achieve your goals.

As you consider which group you are in, think about what prevents you from exercising. Undoubtedly, you know exercise is good for you. Even those people who don't want to admit this know deep down in their subconscious that they should be exercising. So begin to think about why you are not able to do what you know is best. There are so many excuses not to exercise. You've probably heard them all and likely have used several, as have I. So let's dissect what is behind the common habit of making excuses.

An excuse is a reason or an explanation for a behavior. When we make an excuse, we do so because we want to explain why we did not complete a task we think we should have. In the chapters ahead, we will tackle detail regarding why exercise is so vital as well as specific tips to get started and stay with it. To set the groundwork, it is crucial for you to establish your checklist of the excuses that get in your way. Once you acknowledge the excuses you can develop strategies to work past those.

As you go through the list, check off the specific statements that apply to you. (See Appendix A & B for pages you can tear out and post as a reminder to yourself)

- Too busy
- Too tired
- Need to clean the house

- Kids need me to do something
- Too out of shape
- Exercise does not really apply to me, I don't need it
- Will look silly out there
- Don't like to exercise
- To early in the morning
- To late in the day
- Have to work late
- Too cold out
- Too hot out
- Too dark out
- Don't have the right clothes
- Don't have any clean clothes
- Don't have anyone to go with
- My favorite show is on
- Need to answer an email
- Husband wants me to stay home with him
- Not good at it
- Too damn lazy

It is so easy to come up with excuses because they are tangible and very real in terms of the day you are having today. The fact is that women face a huge challenge in juggling multiple aspects of everyday life. There are so many little things that take up the moments right now and get in the way of putting on those exercise shoes and walking out the door. In fact, that first step of getting dressed and going out the door to exercise is the most significant obstacle that we face. Once you close the door behind you, half your work is done albeit the less strenuous half.

So now let's tackle the reasons why you NEED TO exercise. As you read through the subsequent chapters, review this list over and over again to remind yourself why you are changing your ways. Add more reasons that apply personally to you. Check off the reasons you feel exercise should be part of your life:

- Could benefit from losing a few pounds
- Finding it harder to move around because of the extra pounds
- Already have high blood pressure
- Need to lower cholesterol or LDL "the bad cholesterol"
- Could look and feel better if I exercised
- Would be sexier with a few less pounds

- Because my health care provider told me I should
- Favorite clothes don't fit
- Would improve my sex life
- Not sleeping as well as I should
- Am pre-diabetic, diabetic or at risk of this
- Have other health related problems that might improve
- Don't have enough energy
- May inspire my partner to join me
- Need to set a better example for my kids or grandkids
- Am embarrassed by my weight gain
- Am short of breath walking up stairs
- Have a family history of heart disease, diabetes or high blood pressure
- Would feel better about myself
- Really do have enough time
- Would like to meet new people
- May help decrease pain

Now that you have completed your personal list, let's review a few of the complex issues that play into avoidance of doing the right thing, one of the most common being procrastination. Procrastination is defined as; the act of putting off, delay. The reality is that putting things off until later is human nature at least for most people. There are those people who are "Type A" and never procrastinate but most of us do this to some degree. The important thing to appreciate is that the reasons for this behavior are very individual and personal. Some people procrastinate because they work better at the last minute under pressure. Others procrastinate because their "to do" list is filled up with other seemingly important activities. For some, it is the hope that the need to get a certain thing done will go away or that someone else will do it. Procrastination is really just a well-ingrained habit that infiltrates multiple aspects of our lives. Although it is not easy, this habit can be changed with focus and attention to breaking the pattern.

The first steps in changing the habit of procrastination as it relates to your commitment to exercise are to recognize that you are a procrastinator and then to figure out why. You can't begin to work on overcoming the pattern until you consider what your personal reasons are. According to the literature, one core motive for putting things off is fear of failing. A person is afraid that the task will be too difficult and therefore there is no hope of success. They then avoid trying by continually finding a reason to delay. Part of the fear of failing is a lack of confidence, a self-doubt that you can succeed. College students, for example, may procrastinate on their homework out of worry they won't make the grade or that the work will be too hard.

When starting a new activity or exercise there can be the fear that it will be difficult or too tiring. If you start out too vigorously and overdo it, your muscles may be sore and you will hurt every time you move for a few days. Expecting too much of yourself as you begin may lead to disappointment that you can't succeed which just reinforces your failure and self-doubt. The next time you plan to engage in that same activity, you are more likely to find an excuse not do it to thereby intensifying your procrastination.

The other type of fear that leads to procrastination is trepidation of moving out of our comfort zone. Human nature again supports playing things safe by staying with routines that we are used to and comfortable with even when we know change would be a good thing. Consider for example, the attention drawn when breaking out of a peer group to do something new. Even as adults in our fifties, this is not an easy undertaking. Well meaning friends highlight your change by asking questions, making comments and perhaps even teasing. While their intent may be to encourage and support your change, their attention will bring focus to you and could feel awkward. You still are transitioning from your previous comfort zone into something new. Not only will putting on a new outfit which includes spandex or lycra feel foreign, knowing that an exercise routine is going to require hard work and persistence may clearly put you in new territory and out of your comfort zone.

Many type of exercise can raise both these fears in various ways. Joining a class and not being at the level of the other participants carries the risk of perhaps embarrassment or intimidation. There is the fear of not keeping up with others. Maybe you worry that you won't loose any weight or loose it fast enough if that is your goal. Perhaps you worry to some extent about being judged by those around us. Whatever the cause of the fear, your identifying and admitting to this fear will help to chip away at the habit of procrastinating.

As a woman in your late forties or fifties, you can be reassured that these fears while very real are largely unfounded. Our country today is almost in the midst of a health revolution. Everywhere you turn there is information on exercise, diet, the obesity epidemic, the dramatic increase in the incidence of diabetes and other health issues. As a result, there is widespread support for starting a program regardless of your level of fitness. Many class participants include people just like you who have decide to pursue a new adventure. Additionally, the competitiveness that existed when we were younger women seems generally to be gone. Women of our age are much more supportive of their peers and in fact welcoming when another woman joins a group no matter what her size, shape or level of fitness.

If you are a procrastinator, begin to strategize ways to be successful in achieving new goals. In addition to the many tips in the section on strategies, we can discuss here a few which specifically address the issue of procrastination. If fear is causing you to avoid exercising, begin your work out by exercising only for a short amount of time or at a relatively low level of exertion and increase slowly from there. You won't be successful if you try to rush towards the finish and never make it. Use the approach of taking small steps and believe that as long as you are heading in the right direction towards the goal, you are achieving success. Slowly the self-doubt will be replaced by the feeling of accomplishment, which will help you stop procrastinating and keep you motivated to continue your journey.

If you are considering joining a class but procrastinating because of fear of not keeping up, start doing a little bit at home. Get an aerobic stepper and just walk up and down on it. Or go to the library and look for an aerobics tape to begin using at home. There are many available at all levels of fitness so choose one for a beginner. When you start the class you will at least be in shape enough to keep up with the group. Having seen many aerobics classes, it is obvious that there are all levels of people and every participant works at their own pace.

You may be like so many people who procrastination because of the general feeling of not having enough time. It is common to think that exercise will take so much time that it is impossible to carve that out of an already busy schedule. However, if you really look at this excuse, it may be that you are not using your time as efficiently as possible. Sometimes we spend too much time thinking about what we need to do rather than just doing it and by the time we are done thinking about it there really is not enough time.

Perhaps the steps of organizing time differently are all that is necessary to put the needed exercise time into your schedule. Put exercise on the top of your list of things to do for the day. Get that done first especially since it is likely more important to your well being than many other things on your list. Look at what you typically have to accomplish and evaluate where you may be spending time on less valuable things. Let go of certain things that do not have long term benefit.

Consider how many minutes of TV or computer time that you spend each week that could be shifted to exercise time. Or how many minutes of house work or cooking that could be redirected. Your family and friends would probably not even notice the extra dust that would accumulate, the dirty laundry, the unwashed window or the sand on the floor. Post the sign at the end of the book of your door: BEWARE, WOMAN WORKING OUT. ENTER AT YOUR OWN RISK. Or better yet, ask your loved ones or visitors to go for a walk with you and tell them you're leaving the housework for another day. Share your checklists of reasons to exercise to see if you can motivate them. Explain that you would rather not die early with a clean house but would rather have more time to live a full life and die later knowing that you did not care about those few extra crumbs. Think about people you know. How much do you really care how their house looks? Would you rather have your friends and family in your life longer or do you prefer they always keep the house clean? When Erma Bombeck was dying of cancer she wrote that in looking back at her life she wished she had cared less about how her house looked so she could spend more time living.

Find strategies that help you use time more efficiently. One example is that after washing your work out clothes, put everything together right away so you don't have to look for items next time. When it is time to get out, you can just grab what you need rather than wasting valuable time searching. If truly there is not enough time one day, it is OK to shorten the exercise but still do some part of it. Maybe you can't get your thirty-minute walk in but a ten-minute walk is better than no walk. As long as you do not get into the habit of shortening your work out every time, give yourself a break if you need it.

Another example from the excuse list which relates to lack of time is that of having to answer an email. One might say they will go for a walk as soon as they answer an email. The tendency of most people is to sit and answer the email then take a few more minutes to read and answer the few more that just arrived. Next there is a certain web site that you want to look at just for a minute. If you are like me, you then will play a game of solitaire or two since you are sitting right there. Before you know it, all the time you had to walk has been spent on the computer. A strategy to deal with this would be to take the cell phone and rather than replying to the essential email, make a call while you walk. You can then still take care of business and get your exercise done. The person on the other end of the phone might even be impressed that you find it so important to take that walk. If a call rather than an email is not possible, you may also want to consider whether answering the email is as critical as you think or is it just a way for you to procrastinate.

Procrastination may also be a way of coping with pressure either self-imposed or imposed by others. You may consciously or unconsciously sense the enormity of the challenge to get in shape if you feel pressure because you know your behaviors and life style need to change, putting off the hard work may help to alleviate some of the stress you feel. Michele, who I talk about in a later chapter, utilizes a skill in situations like this which she calls "mental gymnastics". An online search of this term links to sites which advocate for mind games and puzzles to keep the brain going. Michele's version of mental gymnastics refers to the practice or habit of mentally spinning around while trying to make a decision or trying to talk yourself into doing or not doing something. It is that cycle of thinking "I should do...... but I can't because of ...... but if I don't then..... but I can do it later.... I definitely will start tomorrow..... and on and on. Then you feel badly about not accomplishing what you meant to do or thought you should whether it is exercise, eat well or other things unrelated to your health. It is like playing mind games with yourself. One of the best ways to step out of the spinning is to stop thinking about it and just do the task. If you can recognize that you are caught in the turmoil of mental gymnastics, you should just stop, choose a direction and move forward. I know it is easier said than done but try it. Next time you start having that mental conversation with yourself, maybe get on your sneakers and take a short brisk walk. Or do a few floor exercises. It will start breaking your cycle and additionally you will feel so much better having completed something you wanted to do.

In the long run, procrastination just creates more pressure because it does not really take care of the underlying problem that needs to be faced. The action of making a decision will relieve some of the pressure. If you are reading this book and feel that you truly cannot fit exercise into your life right now then just accept that decision. Figure out when it will work in your life and make that a goal or objective. Write it down. "Will start exercising on…. (pick a date)". For those of you who admit that you do have the time and are really just procrastinating, try to stop the thinking about what to do. Stop reading for a minute right now and write down your planned date. Make a decision and go with it. This is the first step.

As you consider procrastination, be honest with yourself. If you are a procrastinator, admit it. As mentioned above, putting things off is a common human characteristic. The first step in changing behavior is admitting that it exists. Then you can work on breaking the habit. Go back to your completed check list of excuses and pick a couple to work on that relate specifically to procrastination. Really think of what is behind that excuse for you. Keep that handy as you read the strategies chapter later. Perhaps there are steps along the way you can identify which address a specific excuse of yours.

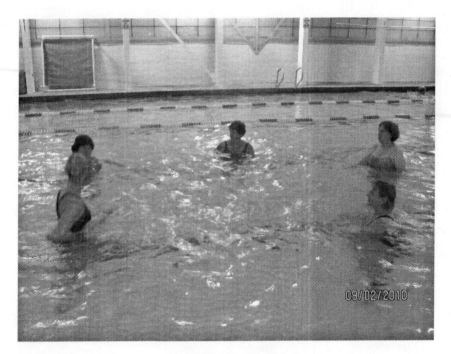

09/02/2010

Water Aerobics class

Chapter 2

SCIENTIFICALLY SPEAKING

Scientific studies evaluating the health benefits of exercise can be found in all areas of printed information including magazines, newspapers and the internet. Television and radio news consistently feature the latest research related to exercise. While each report may focus on a different topic, they all support the well founded fact that staying active positively improves our state of health. Conversely, the science related to inactivity shows that nearly every body system is adversely affected when we are sedentary.

To start with, it is essential to realize that scientific research shows that adhering to an active life style is likely to add years to our lives. There are a multitude of studies supporting this belief. In one recent clinical trial, the investigators evaluated lifetime risk of cardiovascular (heart and blood vessel) disease in men based on fitness levels. The participants in the trial were followed over a long period with an average length of 25 years. The results indicated that men who stayed active had a lower risk of death when compared to men who here inactive. This held true regardless of age, meaning that when active men were compared with inactive men at ages of fifty-five or sixty-five or older the results were consistent. Also the higher level of activity engaged in by participants, the more years that were added to their lives. The results were controlled for additional risk factors for heart disease again validating that the exercise alone was the variable which made the difference. While we cannot say for certain that the findings would be the same for women, it is fairly likely that similar results would be established.

The studies showing that exercise may improve life span are abundant. One that looked at the relationship between fitness levels and the risk of dying found that adults with the lowest fitness level (the least active) were twice as likely to die over the next nine years when compared with those with the next to lowest fitness level. This study did not just look at the older people. It included middle-aged adults like us! This study also found that the number of people in the "most fit group" who died in the follow up period was only six percent compared to twenty five percent in the group with the lowest level of fitness. That is a four times lower rate of early death in those who stayed active! Another surprising finding was that it was not the fitness level throughout life that was most relevant in lowering the death rate. It was recent fitness levels meaning if you have not been an active person all your life or have been less actively recently, it is not too late. Starting exercise at any time will help.

Later chapters will focus more extensively on several specific diseases impacted by life style. There are others not included in this book, such as obstructive sleep apnea, which are well validated by clinical studies. Resources are available at the book store, through your health provider, and on the internet related to areas not covered here.

For now, let's briefly discuss the scientific research which supports the connection between inactivity, a poor diet and the heart. Multiple studies have shown that exercising decreases the risk of plaque buildup in the arteries by lowering the bad components that make up the lipid profile (total cholesterol, LDL, and triglycerides) and increase the good cholesterol (HDL). Exercise will burn up the cholesterol that is traveling around your blood vessels rather than allowing it to be deposited in the vessel walls. A report in the Journal of Lipid Research has shown that adding about an hour of mild exercise each week or a half hour of moderate exercise each week increases the HDL and helps to lessen the LDL and the triglycerides. Although with this small time of exercise the impact may not be huge, every little bit helps.

Think about how minimal this amount of exercise time really is. Take a minute to think of places where you can steal a little time to put towards exercise. If you do something for 10 minutes six days a week or twenty minutes three days a week, you will have completed the one hour of activity. Rather than perusing the throw away magazines that come in the mail, take a quick short walk. Try changing the routine when you get home at the end of the work day. Instead of starting right in on dinner, get out for your exercise. Another routine that works well is when you are starting to feel full at dinner, stop eating, quickly pick up the dishes and get out for a short time. This is a great way to refocus on something much more productive and beneficial, and decrease caloric intake at the same time. Getting up quickly from the table also helps prevent overeating. Once the exercise becomes part of your routine and you feel better, it will move up on your priority list.

Looking at the role of exercise and its impact on diabetes, a recent study found that staying active can delay the onset by several years. Amazingly, in older people, this delay can be as long as 10 years. There was another surprising finding mentioned in this study which corroborates that noted above. The benefits of delaying diabetes is not just demonstrated in a person who has been active their whole life. It was stressed once again that starting an activity program in later years incurs as much benefit as for those who have maintained this lifestyle over many years. Diabetes is discussed in detail in a later chapter however, it is important to reinforce here that the development of diabetes enormously increases the risk of developing significant life changing disabilities and increases death rates.

As women, an issue that we have to deal with is what happens to us as we move into the post-menopausal years. It is a well-known fact that the risk of heart disease goes up after menopause when we lose the protective effect of estrogen. Although the onset of menopause alone increases our risk, the rise in heart disease is more substantial than can be explained by the role of estrogen alone. Researchers have, therefore, been interested in evaluating the other factors which compound the risk of heart disease in the years after menopause.

What they have discovered is that one of the major life style shifts leading to the increase in cardiovascular death rate in post-menopausal women is the rise in the number of obese women. The rate of health problems increased substantially, up to 80 percent according to one study, in women who were obese in middle age. The weight gain is part of the vicious cycle that leads to declining health. The cycle can start with any factor such as menopause leading to weight gain which leads to decrease activity from deconditioning. Following that, there is more weight gain, less exercise and so on. Internally, the vicious cycle is taking its toll through the development of high blood pressure, high cholesterol, changes in the internal world of the blood vessels and diabetes. Exercise is one of the most important factors in preventing or slowing weight gain thereby moderating the development of diseases.

One group of researchers analyzed data from multiple studies looked at the risk of dying based on obesity. The body mass index or BMI (reviewed in a later chapter) was utilized to define level of obesity. The duration of follow up of participants was up to twenty eight years which is extensive for a clinical trial. The results showed that women who were in the higher range of BMI were 13% more likely to die than women in a normal range of BMI. Women in the next highest category of BMI were 44% more likely to die than women in the lower range and in women with the highest BMI, risk of death was increased by 88%. Even more interesting is that given the investigators intent to look solely at the role of obesity, they excluded women with other health problems or risk factors. These findings speak volumes to the importance of weight control to help us live longer.

In addition to all the benefits of exercise to our physical health, there are a multitude of emotional and psychosocial benefits. Many research studies have shown that mood is likely to improve with activity. This fact bears out in all individuals but even more so in those with the lowest level of fitness at the outset. Anxiety and depression are among two of the disorders that have been evaluated in regards to the impact of exercise. While there may be mixed data in the findings from the clinical trials, experts generally agree that improvement in both anxiety and depression through exercise has been supported. Perhaps this is due to the release of hormones known to help improve our mood and outlook; perhaps it is from the feeling of accomplishment or from looking and feeling better. A direct link to the cause of improved mood has not been conclusively determined and to some degree almost does not matter. The important point is the consistently of the research finding that in individuals with mood issues, well-being is improved with exercise.

When we consider other emotional or psychological benefits of exercise, one can't ignore the role of endorphins. Science has shown for years that exercising releases neurohormones which provide an analgesic (pain relieving) and antidepressant effect. The most commonly known neurohormones are the endorphins. Endorphins are a substance in our bodies called polypeptides that are released in response to certain events such as excitement, pain, orgasm and exercise. While it may seem odd to lump those four examples together, each of these create a signal which is transmitted from nerve cells to the spinal cord thereby stimulating the release of endorphins. The "orphan" portion of the word means "a morphine like substance". The release of endorphins provides a natural type of opiate-like pain relief and a natural high. Most people are familiar with the concept of the "runner's high" which is believed to be caused by the release of endorphins. It is important to note here that the endorphin high is not chemically or physiologically similar to the high from ingested opioid drugs such as prescription pain killers and other street drugs like cocaine. The addictive drugs do not pass through the ordinary nervous system pathways that naturally occurring substances travel.

Part of the important role of endorphins is related to the effect on depression. There are a multitude of reasons for feeling down or blue at this stage of our lives. Some of these are further addressed in the chapter on menopause. One important contributing factor is that at this time in life, many women will or already have experienced loss. Depression related to loss, called situation depression, is not uncommon although somewhat under recognized. Finding strategies that help ease the pain of loss is critical to moving forward and finding meaning in life. Aside from loss of loved ones at this time in life, it is reported that some women experience depression simply related to body changes in postmenopausal years. This is a time when we begin to look older as our skin begins to sag, hair may be turning gray, our stomachs bulge and we develop brown spots. If that isn't enough, weight gain may occur simply due to aging. All of this is known to further compound the potential for depression to set in.

Developing a routine of exercise is one effective means to help cope with physical, emotional and social changes that come with loss and to move through the time of change. Add to that an exercise routine with a friend with whom you can share your life events and the transition can be eased at least to some degree.

The scientific literature on the benefits of exercise is unequivocally convincing. As you begin to feel better, realize it is not just your imagination. Even without weight loss, exercise will improve the overall health state of your body. So start now and keep going.

Chapter 3

SAVING YOUR HEART

Just the other day, a thirty nine year old woman, Marion, came in for a cardiac stress test. A couple weeks earlier, she had an episode of chest pressure that was brief and truly did not sound like a heart problem. Just to be on the safe side, she was undergoing a routine exercise stress test. Marion's risk for heart disease was notable including a family history with her mother having had a heart attack at fifty four years old, elevated cholesterol which was not being treated and borderline high blood pressure. Her other risk factor was that she had stopped doing most physical activities aside from that required for daily life and subsequently gained about 20 pounds. Marion indicated that even prior to becoming more sedentary, her weight was higher than it should have been. At this point, she was almost fifty pounds overweight. At six and a half minutes and a hill grade of 12%, she was breathless and could not continue any longer. Overall that is poor exercise capacity for a young woman.

As Marion walked, we talked about her risk for developing a cardiac condition which although she was still fairly young, was on the higher side. As her weight had climbed over the years, so too had her risk. Marion seemed to already know that her fitness ability was low, however, she was unaware that all the factors combined had a huge impact on her heart disease risk and that just by exercising she could improve at least three of these: high blood pressure, high cholesterol, and weight gain. It was obvious that she wanted to be educated and she asked many great questions. After we talked, the hope was that she would become motivated and address her life style to prevent serious negative health events in the future.

The fact that heart disease is the leading cause of death in women and accounts for more deaths than all other major causes of death combined is surprising to many. One out of every three women will develop heart disease in their lifetime compared to one in eight women who will develop breast cancer. And more women die from their heart condition than men. In recent years, there has been a very visible public campaign related to women and breast cancer. Fortunately, this campaign has been very successful with an increase in the awareness of early screening for breast cancer, greater funding for research and improvements in treatment options. The overwhelming success of this public campaign has lead to a decreased in the number of women who die from breast cancer.

Unfortunately, the significant impact of death and disability related to cardiovascular disease in women has been under recognized. A recent published statistic based on polling of women indicated that only 54% of white women are aware of the high rate of death and disability from heart disease. In African American women, Latinos and other ethnic groups, that number is much lower. It is critical to realize that prevention of heart disease will have an enormous impact on saving the lives of women particularly in the post menopausal years. The Go Red for Women campaign, which is sponsored by the American Heart Association, is one major effort focused on raising awareness of heart disease in women.

As you head towards middle age, it is essential to evaluate your risk for the development of heart disease. In fact, with the increasing rate of heart disease in the younger population, this assessment should be done for all adults starting at the age of eighteen. There are studies showing a longitudinal relationship between healthy life style behaviors and longevity. Still, it is never too late to take charge and make changes. Risk factors will be addressed later in the chapter. The first step is to learn what heart disease is and what symptoms might indicate that a problem is emerging.

Cardiovascular disease describes a general category of issues affecting the heart and the other organs and blood vessels throughout the body. This broad grouping can be broken down to diseases affecting the heart, the brain (cerebrovascular disease) and those affecting other blood vessels (peripheral arterial diseases). Diagnoses related to the heart are angina (chest discomfort from reduced blood flow), coronary artery disease (build up of plaque within the arteries of the heart), myocardial infarction or MI (heart attack), and congestive heart failure (difficulty pumping blood out of the heart). High blood pressure and elevated cholesterol can also be considered cardiovascular diseases since they lead to problems which affect the heart. Cholesterol issues are discussed below and there is an entire chapter later in the book devoted to high blood pressure. Let's start with a discussion of the diseases of the heart.

The main physiological process leading to the development of cardiovascular disease is the buildup of fatty substances called plaque within the walls of our arteries. The medical term for this is atherosclerosis. Plaque build up actually starts at the age of two or three with the development of fatty streaks within our vessels. To some degree this is normal. In a reasonably healthy diet, cholesterol substances that are ingested float around in the blood stream and are ordinarily used up or eliminated. As we head into our twenties and have eaten a diet high in fats, excess cholesterol is incorporated into the blood vessel walls and the fatty streaks become more developed. There are a number of additional factors which come into play in the process of plaque development, however generally speaking, if this process continues unabated, the plaque will become significant enough to clog blood vessels and restrict blood flow. In our country as the diet has become less healthy, the blockage from plaque may start even at a younger age. More and more teenagers are being diagnosed with high blood pressure, high cholesterol and diabetes. As mentioned earlier, the accumulation of plaque can happen in any artery in the body. When this occurs in the heart it is referred to as coronary artery disease.

From National Heart Lung and Blood Institute. www.Nhlbi.org

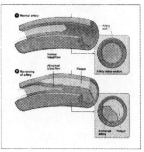

   In addition to the problem of limited blood flow, the plaque may rupture causing the contents of the plaque to spill into the blood vessel itself. The protective mechanisms in our body sense this as a wounded area and want to fix it. Substances are sent in to heal the wound just as they would if you cut your skin. The problem is that this can result in the development of a clot that completely blocks the artery. Whether it is a plaque or a clot that prevents blood from getting past the area, there is no blood flow down stream. The tissues and cells beyond the blockage are unable to receive the essential blood and oxygen needed and if the blood flow is not restored, cells can die.

   The important blood vessels serving the heart are called the coronary arteries. There are three main coronary arteries and multiple branches off these arteries, each of which supply certain areas of the heart muscle. One of the main determinants of how much blood is needed at any given time is the workload and demand that is being placed on the heart. When we are at rest such as during sleep or low level activities, the demand for blood is rather low. However the need for more blood increases when we exercise or are under emotional stress and the arteries must be able to increase the supply of blood to the heart muscle. Coronary arteries that are healthy are able to open up or dilate to bring the increased blood to the heart muscle. When an artery is diseased with plaque it cannot dilate enough to deliver the required blood and the heart cells will be affected. The initial stage of this is lack of blood and oxygen which is called ischemia. If blood flow is not restored, cells become injured and are on their way to dying.

   The classic symptom when cells are not getting enough blood is chest discomfort, pressure or tightness, which is called angina. There are many people who have less classic symptoms so it is important to be aware of these. In addition to sensation in the chest, angina can also cause discomfort in the neck, throat, jaw, teeth, and arms (more commonly the left but either arm). Other symptoms include shortness of breath, pain in the back and often in women there may just be a sense of overwhelming fatigue. The symptoms occur because heart cells are basically screaming for blood and oxygen. Should the vessel be completely blocked such that it is not possible to increase the supply of blood, a heart attack may occur.

When a person experiences anginal symptoms with exercise, if they stop what they are doing, the pressure or discomfort should resolve fairly quickly. Then when exerting again, the symptoms come back. This is a classic pattern indicating a problem with the blood flow to the heart muscle. Alternatively, if the supply can be increased, the flow is restored and the heart will be happy again. One measure to increase supply is taking a commonly used medication like nitroglycerin that opens the coronary arteries to bring more blood to the area. Nitroglycerin also reduces the work load on the heart, decreasing the demand for blood and oxygen. Increasing supply along with decreasing demand reestablishes the balance and the discomfort should resolve. If you experience any of these symptoms with exercise, it is essential to seek an evaluation as soon as possible. Your health care provider may recommend tests to see if there is a blockage in your arteries and if there is a problem, the treatment options will be discussed with you before a heart attack occurs.

It is important to understand that if symptoms of discomfort, pressure or shortness of breath continue despite stopping activities, this is an emergency situation

As noted above, a myocardial infarction or heart attack occurs when there is total blockage and no flow is available to feed the heart muscle. When a person is having a heart attack, cells in the heart are dying. Once dead, scar tissue forms and the affected heart muscle does not participate in the important role of pumping blood around to the rest of the body. When a heart attack victim is identified, restoring blood as quickly as possible is the primary goal. A person should get to the hospital immediately when suffering a heart attack since the less time it takes to reestablish the critical blood supply; the more heart muscle is saved. A common saying to stress the importance of seeking early treatment in this circumstance is "time is muscle".

Sadly, women are more likely to die from a heart attack than men. There are several factors contributing to this, one being that our blood vessels are smaller than men's thereby even further limiting available blood. Women may also have more vague symptoms than men so it is often not as obvious that the symptoms are heart related. Additionally, despite many advances, it continues to be an unfortunate fact that women are not always treated as aggressively as men. We must therefore take charge of our health and wellbeing by preventing cardiovascular disease and by knowing when to seek help.

When blockage is to the point that blood flow is affected, there are several treatment options. One is a fairly common procedure called an angioplasty (PTCA). This procedure increases the blood supply to the heart by inflating a balloon at the site of the plaque thereby breaking the lesion apart. At the time of angioplasty, a small coil, called a stent may be placed in the artery to keep that area open. Cardiac surgery is another option available to bypass clogged areas in coronary arteries and reestablish blood flow below the blockage. An angioplasty, stent or cardiac bypass surgery will treat a specific area but it does not treat the underlying problem that lead to the plaque buildup in the first place. That is where life style modification comes in to prevent further development or worsening of existing plaque. If you are lucky enough be free of narrowed vessels at this point in time, life style modification will help keep your blood vessels healthy for years to come.

While this book is really focused on women, men are affected at a young age even more often than women. Recently, I was once again reminded of the vulnerability of us all, even at a young age. A thirty one year old guy was sent to us for a routine stress test. He had no known significant risk factors aside from family history with his father having a heart attack in his fifties. He worked hard at a moderately active job but did not engage in any routine exercise. He also had a prior history of smoking, having quit two years ago.

After only four minutes of walking on the treadmill, his electrocardiogram (EKG) started showing changes suggesting a blocked artery. Within another minute, he developed the symptom he had initially complained of which was tightness in his throat area, and the EKG changes became more significant and worrisome. The test was stopped and arrangements were made for him to immediately undergo a cardiac catheterization procedure. The test showed that he had barely a thread of a blood flow in an artery which feeds a major and important part of the heart. This was successfully opened with a balloon followed by placement of a stent. The importance of this story is to illustrate that none of us at any age are immune to the development of heart disease. Fortunately, this patient never suffered heart damage and has come to understand the importance of life style modification.

Now that we have discussed the issues with the development of plaque in the coronary arteries, let's move on to how the legs are affected. In the same way that plaque affects the heart, narrowing or blockage in the vessels in the legs leads to poor circulation in the area supplied beyond the plaque. The cells do not receive enough blood and the result is leg pain or fatigue especially with walking. This is called claudication. The most common characteristic of claudication is that whenever a person walks a certain distance the leg pain starts and when the activity is stopped and circulation is restored, the pain will resolve. The person can then walk again but pain will recur after walking a predictable distance. This is the same process we talked about with angina in the heart; the blood supply is inadequate to meet the demand for blood and oxygen in the lower legs. It is basically angina or ischemia to the lower legs and feet. Again, it is the supply-demand ratio causing or relieving the pain.

Ischemia of the legs is not going to kill a person. The main problem, however, is that the area below the blockage is susceptible to tissue breakdown from lack of circulation. Nutrients in the blood and especially oxygen are limited in reaching tissues and cells. Should a wound occur, healing is difficult. There are treatment options available similar to those described for the heart including angioplasty and bypass surgery. Still, the unfortunate outcome may be the need for an amputation if healing is not possible.

The last category mentioned earlier is cerebrovascular disease which refers to atherosclerosis of blood vessels supplying the brain. The most devastating complication from blockage in cerebral vessels is stroke. Again, the process of plaque accumulation in the heart and the legs described earlier mimics how the brain is affected by lack of blood flow. Cells devoid of blood and oxygen die leading to permanent dysfunction. There is further discussion of cerebrovascular disease and stroke in the chapter on high blood pressure.

The first step in decreasing the likelihood of developing cardiovascular disease is to understand your individual risk. Risk factors for cardiovascular disease are broken down into modifiable and nonmodifiable factors. The nonmodifiable ones are those that you cannot change and include sex, age, race, and family history. Men are at increased risk of heart disease compared to women of equal age, however after menopause women catch up. Estrogen has a beneficial effect in preventing build up of plaque in our vessels so when estrogen levels decrease our risk increases. Age is considered a risk factor in men when they reach fifty-five years old and for women it is sixty-five years.

Like age or sex, family history is obviously, not something that can be changed. Having an immediate family member who had heart disease at a young age often means your risk of coronary artery disease is higher. Of course if the family member who had heart disease was an overweight smoker with high blood pressure and diabetes, perhaps the cause of their heart disease was more life style than genes. Still there may be an additional element of genetics that brought on their disease at a younger age. This does not mean that if your father had a heart attack at age 58, your risk is not increased. The age range is just a guideline.

The way in which age is a risk factor for heart disease is not completely understood and continues to be of ongoing interest to researchers. As mentioned earlier, changes are occurring in the heart and other blood vessels starting at the young age of twenty and even younger in obese, inactive teenagers. The heart is a hard working muscle which beats on average 60-80 times a minute, every hour of every day. This calculates to the amazing number of 85,000 to 115,000 times a day. That is in the range of three to four million times a year. Any factor, such as high blood pressure, high cholesterol or weight gain, which adds stress or strain to the heart, will cause it to tire out more quickly. As the coronary arteries age, there is a thickening of the inner layer of the arteries contributing to the stiffening of the blood vessels as well as the plaque build up already discussed. In addition, other substances that are beneficial to blood vessel health become less abundant. Without even considering poor health habits, our bodies are aging independently. It is because of this normal internal aging, that it is so important for us to pay attention to our cardiovascular health. Leading a healthy lifestyle can slow the progression of arterial narrowing and thereby decrease our risk of coronary artery disease.

Modifiable risk factors for cardiovascular disease are those that we can do something to change and include smoking, elevated lipid levels (cholesterol and other components), excess weight, diabetes, low level of physical activity, and high blood pressure. Refer to the checklist at the end of this chapter and in Appendix C to identify your specific risk factors.

Smoking is rather straightforward and not a topic that will be discussed in much detail in this book. If you are currently smoking you are damaging your heart, lungs, blood vessels and obviously yourself. Smoking causes blood vessels to narrow which makes the heart work even harder to pump blood to feed the body. In addition, the chemicals in tobacco products damage the inner lining of the blood vessels. This all contributes to the development of heart disease.

There is no good advice to give other than that you must quit. I know that is easier said than done but every day there are people who quit smoking so it is possible. Research has shown that people who utilize multiple avenues to assist in smoking cessation are more likely to be successful than those who only use one type of resource. For example, going to a smoking cessation class and starting a medication at the same time, yields a higher success rate than either one of these alone. There are now more medications on the market that have been shown to improve success rates than even a few years ago. As a health care provider, we are encouraged to discuss smoking cessation with our patients every time we have a visit. This is not to harass you! Rather, by mentioning this as often as possible, there may be one time that the message hits home and starts someone on the road to quitting. There are multiple resources available to help at any provider's office, on the internet or in any health care facility.

If you do smoke and have not been successful in quitting, it does not mean you should not still commit to other healthy life style behaviors. Clinical studies demonstrate that the most important factors in living a healthy life style are to avoid smoking, follow a balanced nutritious diet, exercise regularly and loose weight if needed. If you only do one of these, you still benefit and for each good habit you add, the benefit increases. Sticking to all four of these healthy habits, decreases risk by a substantial amount each year. It is important to understand, however, that smoking is probably the most significant cardiovascular risk factor of all.

There is a little story I tell patients that exemplifies the difficultly with quitting smoking and the reality that it can be done. Years ago, I was caring for a woman with heart disease in the intensive care unit. She also had a prior history of illicit drug use. When discussing with her the importance of quitting smoking she said "Honey, I have quit cocaine, I have quit narcotic addiction and I have quit alcohol. But I have never found anything harder than trying to quit cigarettes". I learned from her that being sympathetic to the struggle faced by a smoker helps them to know we are not just lecturing for the sake of it, but more so because of the overwhelming concern for the havoc that smoking ravages on the body.

Diabetes and how it relates to cardiovascular disease is reviewed in Chapter 5 in more detail. The most important thing to mention here is that while diabetes is a disease related to insulin secretion and blood sugar control, the fact is that elevation in blood sugar is harmful to blood vessels throughout the entire body. This is especially true when it comes to the small arteries such as those in the heart. About one half to two thirds of people who have diabetes will die from heart disease. Keeping blood sugar in good control does not entirely eliminate the consequence of diabetes, but it does decrease the risk substantially.

The next step in evaluating your risk for coronary artery disease is to understand your personal numbers of cholesterol and other lipid components. In the past, we tended to focus on just the cholesterol however, to really understand your risk; it is important to examine all the values measured in a lipid panel. This includes the total cholesterol, low density lipoprotein (called the LDL or bad cholesterol), the high density lipoprotein (called the HDL or good cholesterol), and the triglyceride level. There are additional sub-fractions of the lipid panel but we will not be discussing those as the four components noted above are the values most commonly assessed.

Cholesterol is a naturally occurring component of the blood that is made by the liver. It is used by our body to make steroid hormones, bile salts which help to digest foods, and it is a part of the outer wall or membrane of our cells. The cholesterol level in our blood is the result of the amount produced by the liver and of the number of saturated fats in our diet. An excessive amount of fats leads to a down regulation of the receptors responsible for effectively removing cholesterol from our blood. The result is an increase in the overall cholesterol levels. Total cholesterol is made up of the total cholesterol in our blood, plus the cholesterol contained in the lipoprotein molecules (in the HDL and LDL).

There are a few genetic disorders present in only a small percent of the population that cause the cholesterol level to elevate. Discussion of this type of high cholesterol is beyond the scope of this book. Individuals with these disorders typically require medications to keep their lipid levels low enough to avoid plaque build up. For people in this group, specialty care with a provider who is an expert in lipid disorder treatment is essential. Treatment should begin in childhood.

For the rest of us, a diet high in saturated and trans fats is the major reason for elevated cholesterol levels underscoring the importance of reviewing your personal intake of these foods. There are guidelines developed through the National Heart Lung and Blood Institute that provide target levels for the individual components of the lipid panel. These are well accepted and guide health care providers in the evaluation of whether or not a person has elevated lipid levels. You can read further about these guidelines by going to the NHLBI web site (www.nhlbi.org) and searching for the guidelines on the Detection, Evaluation and Treatment of High Blood Cholesterol in Adults. Another great resource on this topic is the National Cholesterol Education Program (NCEP). Interestingly, as the scientific guidelines have been revised over the years, the acceptable LDL and triglyceride level has come down while the target HDL has gone up. It would not be surprising in the future to see the recommended numbers to be even lower than the current values.

The factor usually reported first in a lipid panel is the total cholesterol. This number should be no higher than 200mg/dl and lower is better to a certain point. The next number to look at is the low density lipoprotein or LDL (the bad cholesterol). In the last revision of the Guidelines, it was suggested that the LDL should be the primary target of therapies to reduce the risk of plaque build up in our arteries. There are a multitude of scientific clinical trials that have shown that an elevated LDL increases risk for the development of cardiovascular problems. With the recent guideline revision, the acceptable level of LDL was lowered fairly significantly and it is now suggested that ideal LDL in the general population, should be less than 100mg/dl. If a person has known heart disease or other major risk factors, their target is even lower at 70mg/dl.

The high density lipoprotein or HDL (good cholesterol) is another value measured on the lipid profile. The HDL level should be above 40mg/dl at a minimum and most authorities agree that in women the HDL target is 60mg/dl. Research has shown that the higher the HDL, the lower the risk of heart disease and an HDL level higher than 60 is considered to be protective to the heart. In fact the relationship is linear meaning that the longer a person has a high HDL, the longer they are likely to be free of heart disease. Although there has been much research devoted to developing medications that can raise the HDL, there are currently a limited number of drugs available that are helpful in this regard.

The most effective way to raise the HDL is by exercise although if the HDL is very low even exercise may not help. For smokers, quitting may substantially raise the HDL level. Even if the total cholesterol does not change dramatically with risk factor modification, changing the values by lower the LDL and raising the HDL will incur some protection to the heart and other blood vessel systems. Staying engaged in a healthy life style though exercise, maintaining a stable weight and eating right, can lower the lipid profile numbers to an acceptable range. The chapter on diet provides a detailed discussion on foods that affect the lipid profile.

One reality women must face is that as we go through menopause and estrogen declines, LDL and triglycerides tend to rise while the HDL drops. Unfortunately, this can happen despite doing all the right things. Should it be necessary, there are many medications available to lower total cholesterol, LDL and the triglyceride level. Statins are the most commonly known and most frequently used medications to help reach target numbers but there are many other medications which can help. When discussing lipids with patients we see, it is not uncommon for someone to say that they don't like to take medications or they read the side effects and decided not to start them. My response is that side effects are usually reversible with discontinuation of the medications and in fact most people are not troubled by side effects at all. Generally speaking however, the plaque build up in the arteries is going to cause problems long before the side effects ever do. No one likes to take medication but letting the numbers stay high over a long period of time will continue to put one at risk of a blockage in an artery of the heart or elsewhere.

Many people when asked, state that their cholesterol is "pretty good" or "borderline" or "diet controlled". They may even know what their total cholesterol number is. However, when I ask what their LDL and HDL level is not only do they not know their numbers; they do not know why it matters. Without knowing all the values in your lipid panel, you really don't know how well controlled your cholesterol is. Although the responsibility for that knowledge lies with the individual, health care providers need to be more active in educating their patients about what this all really means. I always talk about the importance of "Knowing Your Numbers" (see Appendix F for a usable tool). A person who is active in managing their health care will discuss exactly what the numbers are compared to where they should be with their Primary Care Provider. You can start taking charge of your health by asking for these details. At your next visit with a health care provider ask for a print out of your lipid panel. Keep this so you can see how changes you make affect your levels.

As mentioned earlier, as a Cardiac Nurse Practitioner, I perform stress tests including both regular exercise tests and imaging stress tests. A stress test is done to look for symptoms or electrocardiographic (EKG) changes that might indicate a problem with blood flow to the heart muscle. A routine stress test is simply when a person walks on a treadmill for as long as they can while the EKG is monitored. Our goal is to have someone exercise to at least 85% of his or her age predicted heart rate so we know we have stressed the heart. During this test we are looking for changes on the EKG that indicate narrowing of a coronary artery. We also want to see if a person has any symptoms of angina when the heart is stressed.

With an imaging stress test, one still walks on the treadmill, however in addition to that; pictures are taken of the heart before and after exercise using a radioactive substance. The purpose of this type of stress test is to see if there is a difference in how the heart fills with blood when stressed with exercise compared to the blood flow at rest. The heart muscle lights up from the radioactive tracer. We are looking to evaluate the supply-demand balance that was mentioned earlier. There is a higher demand placed on the heart during exercise and if a blockage is present, blood cannot get through the blockages into the heart muscle. If there is a blockage or narrowing in the coronary arteries, the heart muscle will not take up as much of the radioactive tracer when they exercise.

One of the things that I find concerning as I perform stress tests is how deconditioned many people are. Often they cannot walk more than a few minutes on a treadmill. Granted we do include an uphill grade so we can get the heart rate up fast enough to allow us time to complete many tests in a day, but we do not expect people to start very fast and the hill is not all that steep. The protocol we use starts at 1.7 miles an hour at a ten percent incline. Every three minutes the speed and incline increase until the patient is unable to continue or significant symptoms develop.

When a stress test is performed, we also evaluate functional capacity, which is a person's ability to exercise compared to others of his or her age. If a person in the fifties cannot perform for more than six minutes, that means they are unable to walk up a hill at a pace of 2.5 miles an hour. This would be considered poor functional capacity. It may seem like it is not a big deal to have a diminished functional capacity, however we know that for each minute further a person can walk, cardiovascular risk is decreased by a substantial amount. Functional capacity also correlates with how long a person is likely to live. The higher functional capacity one has, the more likely they are to live longer than a person of the same age with reduced functioning.

You may be thinking that I am talking about older people who cannot walk very long or fast, but that is just not so. Every day I see people of forty, fifty and sixty who are unable to do this test without a significant struggle. Many do not even want to try walking and opt for a chemical test which simulates exercise. This can be a more unpleasant test, yet people would rather go through that than walk for a short time on a treadmill. The other thought you may have is that if we are evaluating for heart disease maybe that is the reason the individual cannot exercise. Very often, the tests on these younger people are screening type tests and there is no significant heart disease present. The decrease in the ability to walk is often related to deconditioning from a sedentary life style and excess weight.

At the same time, there are many days when we have a man or woman near or in their eighties who does better than everyone younger than them. The common finding is that these older people have continued to be active throughout their lives. Many of them take a daily walk or do a variety of other physical activities. Many of these people still work, garden, care for grandkids, volunteer or do something else to keep going. Surprisingly, often times the older person will apologize for not being able to walk longer. We always reassure them that they have done a fabulous job and I generally tell them they beat all the younger people from the day. Recently, one of the women I saw was in her mid-eighties. I asked her what she had done to be so healthy and she said "I just keep moving".

As an aside, many of the older folks tell us their kids want them to slow down, retire, or give up their many activities. We always tell them DON'T DO THAT!!!! The reason they make it to eighty years and longer is because they have continued to be active. The younger people who don't do anything active are the ones who won't live long past retirement age.

The other part of what I do when performing a stress test is to talk about risk factor modification. Surprisingly, there are those people who don't want to hear what they need to do to improve their health. Fortunately though, there are still some who are open-minded and appreciate the advice. They express the need and desire to do more because they realize what terrible shape they are in. In fact, it is not uncommon for someone to tell us that poor performance on a stress test has motivated them to get out more. Whether or not they do get back to exercise, I never know. It is hopeful, at least, when a person recognizes the need and is willing to express that.

Use the checklist below to determine your risk factors for heart disease. This will give you a starting point to determine areas where you can make changes. There is a resource available at www.americanheart.org to help calculate your annual risk of heart disease. In the search area, put in *heart attack risk assessment*. This tool is a great way to see an actual number for your ten year risk of having a heart attack. Then once you have taken charge of the areas where you need to improve your life style, redo the risk calculator. It is a way to positively reinforce that what you are doing really matters.

HEART DISEASE RISK FACTOR CHECKLIST
See appendix C for a tear out copy
Nonmodifiable risk factors:

- Age, post menopausal
- Family History
- Man
- Race (higher risk in African Americans, Mexican Americans, American Indians native Hawaiians and some Asian Americans)

Modifiable risk factors:

- Diabetes
- High blood pressure
- High cholesterol or high number of low density lipoprotein (LDL)
- Low number of the high density lipoprotein
- Over weight or obese
- Inactivity
- Smoking

Chapter 4

LAURIE'S STORY

Laurie and I first met when I was preparing her for discharge after a three day hospital stay. Laurie looked scared. Her wide open eyes and trembling lip gave away her insecurity about leaving the hospital after having suffered a heart attack. She had been admitted with chest pain and was brought urgently to the cardiac catheterization laboratory where a stent was placed to open one of her main arteries. Laurie was fifty years old and never imagined she would end up with this.

As she told me her story, I could see that like so many patients she was still overwhelmed with the events of these three days. Laurie was a school teacher home for the day doing her usual housework. It had started as a minor ache in the center of her chest and gradually the discomfort built until she felt a very heavy pressure all across her mid chest. Fortunately, she had the sense to realize that something was wrong and she asked her oldest son, then ten year olds, to call for help. She lay down on the kitchen floor and listened as he told the 911 operator that his Mom needed an ambulance. Laurie thought she might be having a heart attack.

On the ride to the hospital, the paramedics obtained an electrocardiogram then seeing it was abnormal, they contacted the Emergency Department to alert them to activate the Cardiac Catheterization Laboratory. Hospitals all across the country have time goals they strive to meet in regards to how quickly a patient is treated so early notification is crucial. When an artery is blocked, opening it as quickly as possible saves heart muscle and cells from dying. In Laurie's case it was day time therefore, the staff were already there. A planned non-urgent case was put off as they prepared the lab and when Laurie arrived, they immediately went to work. She was found to have a blockage in her right coronary artery which was easily treated with a balloon and then a stent was placed to keep the vessel open. The damage to her heart was minimal largely due to the fact that she had not ignored her symptoms and had come to the hospital so quickly. Her physical recovery went very well with no problems developing over the next two days. But now that it was time to go home, the emotional impact of the events were hitting her hard.

Laurie had no previous significant health issues however; she did have some warnings and several risk factors. Firstly, her family history of premature heart disease was fairly impressive with five of her eight siblings having some type of cardiac event before the age of 55. One of her brothers had actually died from a heart attack in his forties and her Dad had died young from heart disease. Another sibling had cerebrovascular disease and had undergone a procedure to remove the plaque from her carotid artery. Laurie also had moderately elevated levels of cholesterol and LDL that she had been trying to manage with diet and exercise. She also knew she needed to loose weight as she was about 50 pounds higher than what was desirable. Her day was fairly active, yet it did not include any routine exercise. Laurie admitted in retrospect that her commitment to changing her life style had been somewhat intermittent.

One interesting factor Laurie talked about was that several months earlier at a dentist visit, her blood pressure was found to be elevated. During several subsequent appointments with her primary care provider her blood pressure was often noted to be in the range of 150/80 or higher. It was suggested that she may have "white coat hypertension", a commonly used phrase to mean that people become anxious when their blood pressure is being checked by a health care provider and therefore is higher than it otherwise would be. Many providers feel that white coat hypertension does not require treatment. There is another school of thought that if the blood pressure becomes elevated in this circumstance, there are likely other times of stress throughout every day when the blood pressure is going up so perhaps treatment should, in fact, be initiated. The other explanation given for her elevated blood pressure was that she suffered from anxiety. Unfortunately, it is not uncommon for women to be labeled in this way. In hind sight, Laurie feels that with her high risk factor profile, treatment should have been initiated earlier and more aggressively. She is the first to admit it may not have made a difference in preventing her heart attack. At the same time, given her known high risk, she still wonders.

There was some good news in evaluating her total risk and areas requiring focused life style modification. She did not have diabetes and had never been a smoker. Despite that, when entering her information into a few risk calculators, Laurie's risk of heart disease was 3-4 % not taking into account her significant family history. She did say she now realizes that despite being an educated person, an internet user and someone who paid attention to the news around her, she was fairly uneducated about heart disease and her risk.

About a month after her heart attack, Laurie started attending cardiac rehabilitation which is a monitored exercise and educational program to help people recover and make the necessary changes to take control of their health. Before rehab she was afraid to do anything. Without the program she would still be holding back in many aspects of life out of fear that the chest discomfort would come again. She stated that "I would still be treating myself as an invalid".

Now that 6 months have gone by, Laurie is back to living life fully with no ongoing physical problems. She has lost 20 pounds and is working on shedding still more. Her weekly routine includes walking as often as possible which she not only does for her health but said "I do it for my kids". When she misses a day of her exercise, she tries not to let it stress her out and tells herself "so be it". Laurie did stress that a person in her shoes can't fall into the trap of excusing healthy routines more than a day here or there. Routine activity is not an option any longer, it is essential for her to find time in her busy life. She knows her life and health depend on doing the right things. She also is watching her diet closely and taking her daily medications several of which will be life long.

Several friends and co-workers have taken her experience very seriously and sought a health evaluation for themselves. Laurie talked about how easy it is to pay attention to the little things that mount up to create a big event like her heart attack. She encourages her friends to treat their high blood pressure, elevated cholesterol and extra weight now while they can and before they have to go through the trauma she did. Laurie talked about how simple it is to know your risk.

There are still emotional hurtles that she and her family are working on overcoming. Laurie said when she stops to think about it, "I still can't believe what happened. It all was incredibly scary and surreal." She is so thankful that there was little permanent damage and life is back to its normal hectic pace. A few months after her event, Laurie had a chance to go away to a teacher workshop but her son, now eleven, asked her to please stay home. He does not completely understand all of what happened that day in the kitchen. He does clearly remember the intense fright as he watched his mother being wheeled out to the ambulance and not coming home for a few days. Laurie knows that she looks the same on the outside but on the inside so much has changed.

Chapter 5

HIGH BLOOD PRESSURE

High blood pressure, also known as hypertension (HTN), is sometimes called the "silent killer". The reason it is a silent killer is that a person can have high blood pressure for a long time without any symptoms yet the vital organs (the brain, heart, kidneys and blood vessels) are slowly breaking down due to the constant wear and tear on them from the blood pressure being too high.

To better understand why hypertension adversely affects our bodies, one needs to understand what blood pressure is. The definition of blood pressure is: the force or pressure exerted on the inner walls of the blood vessels when the heart pumps blood around the body. Blood pressure is basically the pressure within the "tank" or the reservoir of the blood vessels. This pressure creates a force that the heart has to work against to push the blood out to feed the rest of the body.

There are two components that make up the blood pressure. The top number or systolic pressure reflects the pressure when the heart is pumping blood out. The bottom number or diastolic pressure is the pressure within the blood vessels when they are relaxed. When the pressure is high, the heart has to work harder to push the blood forward and to move blood around the body. Conversely when the pressure is low, the workload on the heart is much easier.

A detailed document developed by the National Institute of Health called the Seventh Report of the Joint National Committee on the Prevention, Detection, Evaluation and Treatment of High Blood Pressure provides guidelines for management of blood pressure. According to these guidelines, normal blood pressure is when the numbers are less than 120/80. Blood pressure between 120/80 and 140/90 is called the pre-hypertension stage. The is the point at which life style changes may be enough to bring the blood pressure down to prevent true hypertension. Once the blood pressure reaches 140/90 or higher, treatment including medications should be initiated. If a person already has risk factors such as diabetes or heart disease the blood pressure at which medications should be started is a bit lower at 130/85.

This report also indicates that for a blood pressure over 115/75 the risk of cardiovascular disease doubles with each increase of 20/10. That means if your blood pressure is 135/85 your risk of cardiovascular disease is twice as much as if your blood pressure is below 115/75. It is interesting that each time the guidelines have been published and we have more evidence showing the organ damage from high blood pressure, the acceptable numbers are lower than what was previously considered an adequate target. Since a blood pressure value between 120/80 and 140/90 is considered prehypertensive, or the stage before hypertension is established, I always wonder why one would shoot for a blood pressure reading that is considered prehypertensive when the value of 120/80 is considered normal. It is clearly known that a lower blood pressure is better for our health.

A common misconception is that low blood pressure is not good. This is true if the blood pressure is so low that a person has symptoms such as lightheadedness, dizziness or excessive fatigue. However, a low blood pressure means that the heart can do its work very easily. Low blood pressure generally is fine as long as a person feels well, has no symptoms of low blood pressure, and there is not a medical problem causing the low blood pressure.

The cause of high blood pressure is actually not known. We do know that as we age our blood vessels stiffen to some degree. Most people who live long enough will have some degree of high blood pressure. In a much older person, the target blood pressure numbers are not quite as low as for a younger person. Think of an 85 year old with a blood pressure of 146/88. That would be considered hypertension in a fifty year old. But the 85 year old has been doing something right all their life to only have the blood pressure this high at that age. Caution must be taken when treating higher blood pressure numbers in an older person since lowering it too much can be problematic.

What we also know are the risk factors that contribute to the development of high blood pressure. It is no surprise that these risk factors are the same ones that contribute to many other chronic diseases such as heart disease, stroke, diabetes, kidney disease and problems with circulation to the legs and feet. Obesity is one of the significant risk factors for the development of high blood pressure and unfortunately with our rising population of obese people, there has been a significant rise in individuals with high blood pressure. Some estimates suggest that more than 40% of obese individuals also have hypertension.

Other risk factors for high blood pressure include:
- Smoking
- Inactivity
- Too much salt in the diet
- Stress
- Older age
- Excess alcohol
- Race: African American, Hispanic American, Asian American, Pacific Islander or American Indian
- Diseases of the kidneys, adrenal glands and thyroid

As previously mentioned, one of the significant problems with high blood pressure is that many people are not aware that they have it because early on there are no symptoms. Eventually, the vulnerable organs are affected and symptoms appear such as a stroke, renal failure or heart failure. The problem is that by the time a person is symptomatic, permanent damage may already be done. This underscores the importance of regular screening for HTN especially as we age. When high blood pressure is identified early, treatment with either life style changes or medication can reverse some of the physiological consequence and prevent disabling problems.

Many people who know their blood pressure is too high go without treatment either because they do not want to take medications or they have not been convinced of the importance of treating this insidious disease. Unfortunately, another reason for untreated hypertension is that health care providers are not as aggressive as they should be. There are a number of reasons for this which are beyond the scope of this book. However, what is reassuring is that there has been slow improvement in the number of treated individuals especially as consumers become more educated about this important risk factor and health care providers learn more about the consequences of untreated HTN.

So, let's discuss the negative effects of long standing untreated high blood pressure in more detail. Blood vessels run throughout our entire body, therefore problems related to integrity of the blood vessels can occur just about anywhere. The health or integrity of the blood vessel walls is increasingly recognized as crucial to our overall well being. Researchers continue to learn that blood vessels are not just tubes to hold and transport blood and other chemical substances. They are highly active organs that carry out many functions such as the release of chemical substances utilized in other parts of the body and the transport of elements from the blood stream into the cells. When the blood vessels are not healthy, a variety of changes occur including increased deposit of fats in the blood vessel walls, the development of resistance to the insulin we need, inflammation and stiffening of the vessels and breakdown in transport mechanisms which are essential for cells to do their work. These changes increase the likelihood of chronic diseases developing.

One area of the body that is significantly affected by high blood pressure is the left ventricle (LV) of the heart. The left ventricle is the pumping chamber of the heart, basically the work horse. The left ventricle is the chamber that forces blood out of the heart through the aortic valve to circulate around the entire body. In order to eject blood, the LV has to generate more pressure than whatever the blood pressure is in order to open the aortic valve and allow blood to be ejected. This is the case every beat, every minute of every day. Since the average heart beats over one hundred thousand times a day that is a lot of work the heart has to do. Imagine if you did that many push up each day or climbed that many stairs. You would have very well-developed arm or leg muscles. The heart muscle becomes larger in the same way from all the extra work that is demanded of it when the blood pressure is high and while that may be good for your arms and legs, it is not good for the heart. A heart muscle that is too large becomes less efficient and cannot pump blood forward as well as it should. The heart muscle also become stiffer which creates problems with its ability to stretch adequately when needed.

Imagine that there is a door (the aortic valve of the heart) that needs to be opened to allow you (the blood) to leave a room. If there are 100 people pushing against the other side of the door, you need to work really hard to open it. That is similar to the work the heart has to do to force open the valve because of the high blood pressure on the other side. If you take away half the people, or in this case lower the blood pressure, you can open the door much more easily. Using this visual analogy, think about how hard the left ventricle has to work when the blood pressure is 160/90 compared to the work it has to do when the pressure is 120/80 or less.

One relatively common cardiac condition that develops as a result of high blood pressure is called diastolic heart failure or the stiff heart described above. Diastolic heart failure does not mean the heart is going to stop working. It means the heart becomes less elastic and can't relax adequately when it should thus making it less efficient in its ability to handle any extra fluid that can build up in the body.

There are several reasons for extra fluid to develop, with a very common one being too much salt in the diet. If you have more salt, the body will hold onto more water to dilute the salt. As a result, the total volume in the blood vessels will go up. This blood will make its way to the heart and the heart has to stretch in order to accept this volume. In diastolic heart failure when the heart is stiff, it can only stretch a certain amount which is less than in a normal heart. The heart can't push the blood forward, and there is no more room in the ventricular chamber, therefore it backs up. The path of least resistance for the blood to go from the left side of the heart is backwards into the lungs. As blood backs up into the lungs, water moves into the air spaces. As you can imagine, water does not belong in the air spaces of our lungs. The resulting symptom is difficulty breathing or shortness of breath.

The shortness of breath that develops because the heart can't push blood forward is a frequent and uncomfortable symptom that causes people to come to the hospital. According to patients, shortness of breath is one of the worst feelings a person can experience and one that we should all be motivated to avoid. Unfortunately, heart failure is a very common condition and a leading cause of hospitalization in our country. The good news is that when a person arrives at the hospital with shortness of breath from too much fluid, it is most often quickly treatable with medication. The bad news is that reversing the stiff heart problem is difficult if not impossible depending on how advanced the damage is. Again, citing the NHLBI report, reduction of blood pressure can lower the risk of heart failure by more than 50 percent. That is a huge effect and one that can actually be accomplished by making small steps towards improved health.

The kidneys are another organ adversely affected by high blood pressure. The physiological factors leading to the decline in kidney function are very complex. As with the heart, the high pressure that the kidneys have to work against causes damage to cells within the working part of the kidneys.

Suffice it to say that the end result is enlargement and stiffening of the filtering unit of the kidney called the glomeruli. These changes prevent the kidneys from doing their critical work of cleaning the blood of substances which we don't need such as electrolytes and other waste products. When these accumulate in the blood stream, cells throughout the entire body are unable to work as efficiently as they should. For example, the kidneys normally maintain potassium in a delicate balance by keeping what we need in the blood and filtering out and excreting what we don't need. All cells rely on potassium to function properly. The heart is particularly sensitive to having the potassium within the normal range and it is not happy when the potassium level is too high or too low. It is actually dangerous to have potassium out of range. When the glomeruli are not working, the potassium level can elevate to a point where it is dangerous for the heart. The same is true for many other substances within our body.

The kidneys have many other functions including keeping fluid in balance, making red blood cells, producing hormones to help regulate other body functions and building bones. All of these can be affected when there is a decline in kidney function. In the early stages of kidney disease, just like with high blood pressure, there are no symptoms. It is when damage is becoming fairly significant and permanent that symptoms will occur.

The high pressure in the kidneys may cause the vital tissue to become inflamed which can lead to impairment of the kidney function and eventually progress to total kidney failure. Our body will compensate for declining kidney function for a while, but if the blood pressure is not brought down, more damage will be done. As mentioned earlier, the risk factors for many chronic diseases including diabetes (discussed in a later chapter) and HTN overlap. The risk of significant damage goes up in people who have both conditions. Add to that any additional health issues such as high cholesterol, obesity and smoking and the negative spiral is only worsened.

Moving away from the kidneys, another problem associated with high blood pressure is the risk of a stroke. The blood vessels in the head are very sensitive to changes from prolonged exposure to high blood pressure. Some of the vessels in the head are very small. When exposed to increased pressure over time, they become stiff and are unable to contract and relax in response to the flow of blood just as described for the other vessels in the body. Eventually the sustained high pressure causes damage to the vessel walls and a rupture occurs. When this happens, there will be bleeding in the brain leading to increased pressure within the skull. Since the skull is a rigid structure and cannot expand, brain tissue is essentially squished by the excess volume of blood. Brain cell function is impaired and a stroke results.

There are different types of stroke and several mechanisms that can cause the stroke to occur. One is rupture and bleeding as already noted. Another type of stroke occurs when plaque builds up in the artery causing narrowing and thereby limiting blood flow to the brain tissue. The vessels in the head become atherosclerotic from the cholesterol levels being too high. This is the identical process that causes a heart attack as was discussed earlier in the chapter on the heart. When this becomes severe enough, a total blockage to blood flow results. When there is no flow beyond the blockage and blood does not get to an area of the brain, the cells and tissue will die. The consequences will be similar to a stroke from bleeding although the actual process leading to the stroke is different.

Our country leads all other countries in the number of people who suffer a stroke due to high blood pressure. That is pretty amazing considering that we reportedly live in one of the wealthiest and most advanced countries in the world. Stroke is one of the major causes of death in our country and also is the leading cause of long term substantial disability. Lowering blood pressure alone could cut the number of strokes by HALF saving several hundred thousand people from the devastation of a disabling or deadly stroke. Again, an amazing statistic especially knowing that lowering the blood pressure is a relatively easy thing to do between life style changes and available medications.

It was stated earlier how overwhelming chronic illness can be to individuals and their families but it must be repeated here. Watching people go through the traumatic life changing impact of stroke is a very humbling experience. Stroke is one of the most overwhelming events that people can experience because of the profound impact of permanent damage. The main consequences of a stroke are loss of ability to use an arm or leg or both, some degree of inability to speak or understand, or loss of part or all of the vision. The worst outcome is a complete loss of functional abilities. People in this state may require complete care for the rest of their lives.

The good news, once again, is that exercise and weight loss can limit or reverse these negative consequences especially if done before the damage is advanced. A long term study by Dr. William Castelli in Framingham, Massachusetts called The Framingham Heart Study has shown that 5 pound weight loss can decrease cardiac risk by 40%. Aerobic exercise can lead to a decrease of up to 10mm in blood pressure. While this does not seem like a considerable amount, the overall health benefit is in fact significant. This may mean the difference between requiring medication for treatment of blood pressure or not. Or for a person on multiple medications for high blood pressure, perhaps one can be eliminated.

Combined with weight loss and exercise, dietary changes such as a reduction in salt intake, will decrease blood pressure even more. In one study called the Dietary Intervention Study in Hypertension groups of people were compared in regards to the impact of dietary changes on blood pressure control. The group required to limit salt intake lowered blood pressure enough to remain off medications. In those whose dietary changes lead to an average weight loss of ten pounds, 60% maintained their weight loss after one year and remained off blood pressure control medications. A very important point in both these studies is that weight loss does not have to be huge to incur an enormous benefit to your health. So if you think you need to loose 50 pounds, go back to the goals and make your initial target smaller. Each pound you shed, lowers the blood pressure, lowers your risks of long term problems, and raises your level of health.

The salt intake in the average American diet is 6-8 grams or 6000-8000 milligrams per day. When a person is afflicted with heart failure, it is recommended that they reduce their salt intake to no more than 2000 milligrams per day. While most people think that getting rid of the salt shaker will bring about a substantial reduction, most of the salt that is consumed is what is present in processed foods. Most foods that are processed in any way have salt added to them. In a later chapter, reading food labels is discussed. Start educating yourself now by reviewing the food labels of common items in your diet.

The Federal Government through its research on dietary ways to reduce salt intake and thereby lower blood pressure has come up with a diet called the DASH diet. The main recommendations of this diet include lowering salt, eating less processed foods and eating more fresh fruits, vegetables, grains and fresh cooked meats, chicken and fish. Following the DASH diet can lower blood pressure 8-14 points. Coupled with increase activity and weight loss, this simple step may help control blood pressure for a number of years. As noted earlier, we know that the likelihood of developing high blood pressure goes up as we age just from the normal physiological aging process, These fairly simple steps can slow that progression and keep a person healthier for much longer.

Admittedly, there are times when a person is doing all the right things and they still develop hypertension. It may be genetic, due to race, or other physiological issues. That is when medications must be utilized in addition to developing healthy life style behaviors. I can't tell you how often I hear people say they "don't like to take medications". They may not even be taking the ones prescribed in part because they don't understand how essential these medications are. Almost no one likes to take medications. However, what I remind them is that years ago, people did not live as long or as well as they now can because the medications we have were not available years ago. Without treating conditions like high blood pressure, the person who "does not like medications" is playing Russian Roulette with they body. We have an arsenal of medications available today to deal with this condition, often times, with minimal or no side effects. The choice is simple, either start life style modification behaviors that will treat hypertension or take medications. Otherwise, complications are highly likely to develop. There is no middle road and the problem is not going to go away on its own.

Chapter 6

SALLY'S STORY

Sally is a 56 year old Nurse Practitioner who has struggled with her weight for many years. She is one of those people who does the "yo yo" thing, constantly in a flux one way or the other. As a busy person with four girls she raised and now several grandchildren, finding time for herself is often last on her list. Over the years I have known Sally, she has been on one kind of a diet or another. She has done shakes, Weight Watchers, cabbage soup diets, the age old just "watching what you eat diet" and several others. Of course with each, her weight has gone down for a time but when Sally would stop paying attention, the weight would creep back up again.

Sally said she has always had two wardrobe sizes, fluctuating from larger to small and back again. When the weight increases to where she can't fit in the larger size, she starts a new diet. Usually she will then drop back to a comfortable size and often stay there for at least a few months. A few years ago at the crux of an especially difficult time in her personal life, Sally's weight crept up again. Around the same time, she had blood work done as part of her routine yearly physical examination and to no surprise, her cholesterol was elevated at 246mg/dl and her LDL was 106. She was already on a cholesterol lowering drug which had brought her levels down some but clearly not to an acceptable range. When we talked, Sally also mentioned that she was self-conscious counseling cardiac patients about risk factors and healthy behaviors when it was fairly obvious that she was not living what she was teaching.

Sally said "I know I will never be skinny, but I had to get control. At that point I was really short of breath with exertion and I knew it was just from being too heavy". Sally recognized that it was time to get back into the swing of healthier choices both in regards to the food she was eating and her activity level. She knew that without a structured program she would not have the will power to stick with it so she bought into a dietary plan that included prepackaged shakes. For the first four weeks, Sally had to consume 4 shakes a day and was allowed one meal. After that, food was slowly reintroduced with the focus on learning to eat healthy and in moderation. Throughout those weeks the excess weight slowly began to fade away.

Prior to starting the shake package, Sally exercised intermittently and mostly on the weekends. She said "I was a weekend warrior and even then did not exercise every weekend". As part of the program it was recommended to begin an exercise routine so she joined Boot Camp, which has become very popular at most fitness centers. Boot Camp is intended to give you a full body workout utilizing both aerobic activity and muscle building. Four mornings a week, Sally drags herself out of bed at an ungodly hour of 4:30 in the morning to get to class before work. Aside from when she had to take a break for surgery, she has been religious about making it to her class. If she cannot get there in the morning, there are late day classes available which Sally points out, are very crowded. When I asked her how it was to start Boot Camp after not exercising regularly, she said her class is "completely non-competitive and includes people of all ages, sizes, and abilities. I never feel badly when I have to slow down. Some days I am tired or sore so I just do the best I can. Everyone has those days".

With the combination of diet and exercise, the weight continued to drop off and overall she lost 35 pounds. Sally said she has never been at her ideal weight and perhaps never will but still she is very happy with her accomplishments. Overall she feels much better, has more energy and is much stronger. Sally challenged one of her co-workers, also on an exercise program, to a treadmill battle using the protocol we do for stress tests. She was able to complete more than twelve minutes at a sixteen percent incline and could have continued even longer. Months before, she never could have done that well.

Sally also had her lipid panel rechecked and both her total cholesterol and the LDL had dropped substantially. The LDL (bad cholesterol) was now down to 72, which is at the target we work to achieve in people with documented heart disease. Sally knows it is the weight loss and exercise that really made the difference. She had been on a statin when she began her new routine however; she had not been able to lower her numbers to reach acceptable goals until she became serious about her exercise.

Sally said an additional motivation to get her health in order was to be a good role model to her children. Her daughter, Katie, then 24 years old, was struggling with her weight at 60 pounds more than ideal body weight. Sally said Katie held her extra weight mostly in the abdominal region, the type of "blubbery fat" associated with what is called central obesity. It is known that when the weight is more concentrated in this area there is an increased likelihood of metabolic syndrome and diabetes. "I was so worried about her. She was a set up for diabetes and I knew that if she did not take the weight off now it was going to be harder as she got older." Sally encouraged Katie to do the shake program with her and even offered to purchase the package but initially Katie declined. Sally did note that her daughter was somewhat defensive talking about her need to drop pounds, as is common with overweight people. Katie said it felt unhealthy to eat so little food, like she was anorexic. Then Katie realized that her mom was only trying to help her and she was spot-on with her concerns so she eventually took up her offer.

Once Katie got started there was no stopping her. The weight came off quickly in the beginning which often happens when a person has a lot of fat to lose. Then as she realized how much better she was feeling, Katie incorporated running into her day. Now, barely about one year later, she has competed in a half marathon and has lost 60 pounds!! In just a few months from now she will run in the Chicago Marathon. Good luck Katie.

It has been almost a little over a year since Sally decided now was the time to take charge. She still is a bit on the yo yo and occasionally gives in to eating foods she should avoid, but she quickly gets herself back on track when she falls off. When asked what her biggest challenge has been Sally said "I am a social eater. I love to get together with my family and friends and when we are together, we eat. That is just what we like to do. We even compete to see who can make the most delicious food which is of course, usually the worst food with the highest calories". Sally said now that everyone knows she and Katie are working so hard to stay fit, "we are all making an effort".

The advice Sally said to give readers is that "you have to find exercise you like or you just won't do it". She certainly knows, having tried a variety of activities. Boot Camp has been the perfect fit for her and one that she keeps getting up before the crack of dawn to attend. Sally summed things up by saying "I would rather be fifteen pounds lighter but I know I am better off now than I was before starting all this. I just don't have that kind of will power". Still she feels so much better than last year and hopes she never goes back. Now when Sally talks to patients struggling on the treadmill, she is able to share her personal experience with them. She now practices what she preaches.

Chapter 7

SETTING GOALS

Hopefully you are starting to be convinced that increasing your exercise or starting an exercise program is the right thing for you. Intellectually knowing the importance of this is the easy part. As stressed earlier, the hard part is changing your habits, starting an exercise routine and doing that most every day for the rest of your life. Let's not be disillusioned to think making these changes is not a lot of hard work, especially if you have not been active. For those who are overweight or out of shape, it will be uncomfortable particularly in the beginning. You may be out of breath, have sore muscles and feel that you will never improve. So how can you get going and stick with it?

As you start your exercise program, think about what you want to accomplish both in the short term and the long term. The first concrete step you can take is to develop a list of your goals and objectives. Keep that handy so you can refer to your list as a reminder of why you are working so hard. This is especially helpful if you become discouraged or have times when you want to give up. Put your list in an obvious spot as a constant reminder to you and to others in your household. The refrigerator door is a great place.

A goal is defined as: the result of achievement toward which effort is directed; aim; end; the terminal point in the race. The goal is the big outcome that you want to achieve. To get yourself started, think about what your goal is. It may be:

- To feel better
- To loose _____ pounds
- To keep up with husband, friends, children, grandchildren
- To be less short of breath when doing things
- To lower blood pressure
- To cut calories eaten or to burn more calories than what is taken in
- To lower cholesterol
- To fit into some of my old clothes
- To get rid of old clothes and buy new ones in a smaller size
- To spend less money at the fast food restaurants
- To come off some medications
- To have better control of diabetes
- To avoid becoming a diabetic
- To feel better about myself
- Other:_____

The goal may be somewhat immeasurable. It does not have to be terribly specific, perhaps something basic such as such as to feel better. Or it may be a very specific long term desire such as loosing a certain amount of weight. From the goal, the objectives are then developed. An objective is defined as: something that one's efforts or actions are intended to attain or accomplish; a target; purpose. The objectives help you break down the goal into smaller steps. It is measurable and identifies the more specific smaller targets you want to achieve. If you only focus on the goal, you may become discouraged since it may take a long time to get to that end point. The objectives help you appreciate the small steps on your journey. The quote at the start of the book is sort of about goals and objectives: *The journey of a thousand miles begins with one step*. The journey is the goal; each step along the way is the objective.

As an example, let's say you want to loose 30 pounds. That is going to take some time and a fair amount of work. It would be easy to be discouraged as the weeks go by and you are not reaching your goal quickly enough. However if you set an objective of maybe loosing 2 pounds this week by exercising more and eating less, you are more likely to reach that target and less likely to become frustrated and give up. Making your gains smaller so you can see progress will help keep you motivated. Remember as long as you are heading in the right direction, towards your goal, you are doing great.

You can make your objectives a type of checklist or "To Do" list and check or cross off the items as you accomplish them. For those even more organized that this, develop a spread sheet with objectives on one side and weeks at the top. Then start filling it in. Suggested objectives are:

- Walk 3 times this week for 20 minutes each time. Do this for _____ weeks.
- After _____ weeks, walk _____ times for _____ minutes each time (increase amount)
- After _____weeks, do the same walk in _____ less minutes.
- Add _____ miles each week. (make this a small amount like ¼ mile)
- Call the local fitness center and ask about membership fees. Be sure to ask about discounts or trial incentives.
- Find one group program to join. A great place to check is your local hospital. Many have programs that may be less expensive than a fitness center.
- Try a new fitness activity that sounds fun.
- Get a buddy to work out with. Call _____ and make a date.
- Pick a day that you can work out with your friend and plan to do that for the next several weeks. _____ (day)
- Avoid eating _____(list a food) for _____ days
- Loose _____ pounds. Make this a very small number such as 1-3. If you set it too high, you will be discouraged.
- Tell at least one person what your goals and objectives are. This can help you stay motivated especially if it is a person who will check in with you as to how you are doing.
- Skip using the drive up window at the bank, coffee shop, or any other drive up every day this week. Just getting out of the car each time will help you burn calories.
- Choose a parking space half way down the lot every time you do an errand.
- Next week, choose a parking spot at the end of the lot.
- Tell your primary care provider what your health objectives are. Work out specific goals with them in regards to your numbers.

When you don't feel motivated, take out your list. Maybe the first item in your list will be to put on your exercise clothes and walk to the end of the street. Even if you don't go any further than that, it is a start. Read the chapter on the Five Minute Rule before you head out. Take a minute to work on your goals and objectives right now.

There is one other strategy to help in regards to goal setting and keeping you motivated that is particularly effective. There are so many group events like breast cancer walks, Go Red for Women events, and other walks and runs for a variety of causes. Pick one several months from now that you want to enter. Make it one of your goals to complete one of these events. It will give you a target to shoot for and will keep you motivated knowing that you have to get ready for it. Be sure to pay your entry fee early. If you are like many people, you won't want to waste the money by not following through. You might be surprised at how much fun these events can be. The group energy is captivating. I also have found that as we age, much of the competitiveness that exists in younger athletes abates. These events are more about participating and finishing than doing it within a certain amount of time. In the Timberman Triathlon, the people I talked with did not even discuss their finish time. Everyone was thrilled to simply be there.

Last year I walked with my friend Holly in a local fund raising walk/ run event. When we were milling about watching finishers, there was suddenly loud cheering from the crowd. One of the fifty something woman in our town was sprinting full force towards the finish line. Although she was not running fast compared to some of the previous finishers, for her it was a sprint. She told me later that her goal was just to do better than last year by completing the course in under a certain number of minutes. She had enlisted the help of her friend's son to walk with her for the early part of the course knowing that his pace would get her start out faster. When she came up over the final hill and saw the FINISH sign ahead, she started sprinting towards the cheering crowd. What I remember most is the huge smile on her face. No one cared what her time was. It only mattered that she was out there and more importantly had achieved her goal.

So get out that paper and pencil and start writing your goals and objectives. Post them some place that your family members can see them. Talk about what you are doing. It will help you to stick with it. Do let others know that you don't want to be pressured. And don't feel bad if you miss a day or mess up now and then as long as you stay on track. It is fine to take a day off here and there but don't get in the habit of excusing yourself more than one day at a time. Look towards the goal and realize that every step towards that is one step in the right direction. You may not get there fast but as long as you are going forward, you are making progress.

Chapter 8

WEIGHT, EXERCISE AND DIABETES CONNECTION

Your body is an intricately connected network of amazing processes delicately balanced to keep you alive and well. How you care for yourself impacts the balance, shifting from health to risk and finally disease if healthy behaviors are ignored. The association between weight, diabetes, heart disease, high blood pressure, and stroke risk is very complex and dynamic. Researchers are constantly gaining new knowledge about the multifaceted interplay of factors related to diabetes and its effect on the human body, yet, many questions continue to remain unanswered. This chapter will discuss what we know about diabetes and how weight gain may bring about the development of this difficult disease. At the end, it is my hope that readers of this chapter will be even more convinced that it is time to start a routine exercise program and never look back to their old lifestyle.

Diabetes is one of the most threatening diseases that can develop due to poor lifestyle habits. While there are individuals who develop diabetes at a young age due to genetic factors, the primary cause of diabetes is weight gain. You can pick up almost any magazine, newspaper or online publication and read about the explosion of obesity in our country and the resulting fact that diabetes is at epidemic proportions. Some resources suggest that 60% of our population is overweight or obese bringing the number of people inflicted with diabetes to all time high.

Important facts related to diabetes include:

- Diabetes is the 6th leading cause of death in the United States
- 19.3 million people in the United States have diabetes
- Nearly 6 million of those people are undiagnosed which means that diabetes is ravaging their bodies without their awareness
- When those with impaired glucose tolerance is added to the number of diabetics, there are 41 million people afflicted
- Men diagnosed with diabetes may lose more than 11 years of life. Women will lose more than 14 years of life.
- Diabetics are at significantly increased risk of heart disease and heart attacks. About half of the deaths caused by diabetes are because of an issue with the heart
- Type 2 diabetes is the leading cause of end stage kidney disease which often leads to dialysis
- Type 2 diabetes is the leading cause of new cases of blindness
- Individuals with diabetes are at increased risk of stroke with permanent disability
- Diabetes contributes to non-healing of wounds and the development of gangrene leading to limb loss
- Lost productivity due to diabetes is a significant factor in the work force

So what really is diabetes? Many people think diabetes is just a problem with "the blood sugar" or a problem with the pancreas which normally secretes the right amount of insulin to control the blood sugar. While in its simplest form perhaps that is true, it is essential to understand that diabetes is not just a problem with the blood sugar and the pancreas. A more accurate way to describe diabetes is a "micro-vascular" disease affecting the blood vessels throughout the entire body. It is true that the primary measurement for evaluating diabetes is the blood sugar; however a blood sugar that is too high damages the small blood vessels through the body. It is this damage to the blood vessels that leads to the terrible complications of diabetes. More on that later.

Diabetes Mellitus is the medical name for a metabolic disease caused by an imbalance in the manufacture, use and breakdown of glucose (sugar). A Type 1 diabetic is dependent on insulin to control the blood sugar where a Type 2 diabetic can still use pills to help manage their disease although they also may also be on insulin. A young person is more likely to have Type 1 diabetes resulting from impairment of the pancreas to produce insulin. There may be otherwise healthy individuals who are afflicted regardless of life style. Type 2 diabetics typically develop the disease at a later age and more commonly have contributing risk factors.

When a person has diabetes, their body is not able to use food for energy in the same way as a person without diabetes can. Normally when you eat, food is broken down into sugar called glucose. The glucose travels through your blood vessels where insulin is available. Insulin's job is to help the glucose make its way into the cells where it can be used for energy. Insulin comes from the pancreas which of course is why the pancreas is considered to be the failing organ in diabetes. In a diabetic, the insulin is either unavailable or unable to do its usual work thereby allowing the sugar to hang around in the blood. The sugar level in the blood rises beyond normal levels causing symptoms and if sustained, long-term complications result.

Before full-blown diabetes develops, there is often a stage called pre-diabetes or impaired glucose tolerance. This means that either the cells are becoming resistant to the insulin that is produced or that the body cannot produce enough insulin to keep up with the amount of sugar floating around. When you overeat, you are overloading your blood vessels with sugar forcing the pancreas, insulin production and blood cell transport processes to try to keep up. In addition, hormones and peptides are secreted by the stomach and intestines to break down the ingested food. A higher intake of food and certain sugars leads to an increase in the demand for these substances. Eventually, like any consistently overworked system, the process fails, the systems shut down, and the sugar is unable to be processed properly.

Once diabetes has moved beyond the pre-diabetes stage, other physiological factors come into play. Cells become resistant to the action of insulin (called insulin resistance), too much insulin remains in the blood stream (called hyperinsulinemia) and the ability of the cells to take in insulin decreases. It can be confusing to understand because each mechanism affects the other, thereby creating a kind of cyclical interaction or a vicious cycle where there is no end. Impaired glucose tolerance (IGT) occurs between the states of normal glucose metabolism and the onset of true diabetes and is created by this insulin resistance and hyperinsulinemia.

One causative factor for pre-diabetes is excess weight especially in the waist area. The other two important risk factors are hypertension and a lipid profile showing high triglycerides and/or a low HDL. The presence of all three is what is called the metabolic syndrome. A person who has either metabolic syndrome or pre diabetes is at high risk of developing diabetes however, the progression to diabetes can be delayed or even stopped by changing lifestyle, in particular by exercising, changing eating patterns and loosing even a modest amount of weight. The American Diabetes Association suggests a 5-10% reduction in weight may be enough to significantly impact the potential risk. Consider if you weigh 180 pounds and this is too high for you. You only need to loose nine pounds to achieve a 5% weight reduction and lessen your risk of developing diabetes. More weight loss of course would be beneficial yet making this small amount of loss a goal is a great first step.

The diagnosis of diabetes is made by obtaining blood sugar levels. The normal level of blood sugar is below100mg/dl. When the fasting blood sugar result is between 100 to 125mg/dl, a person is considered to be pre-diabetic. A fasting blood sugar obtained on two separate days with a result over 126mg/dl is considered diagnostic for diabetes. A non-fasting blood sugar of 200mg/dl is suggestive of diabetes and should be evaluated further with additional tests.

The other test to evaluate for diabetes is called the hemoglobin A1C (HbA1c). Rather than providing a number of what the blood sugar level is at the time the blood is obtained, the HbA1c tells what the blood sugar average has been over six to twelve weeks. This number should be below 6.0 in people who do not have diabetes. A value greater than 6.5 should be rechecked, however a second test with a similar result confirms that diabetes is present. These numbers are accepted as standard for the general population, however keep in mind that there are additional elements and values that a health care provider will consider in establishing a definitive diagnosis.

Additional mechanisms by which diabetes develops in individuals who are overweight is continually of interest to researchers, however, there are some aspect that are at least partially understood. Basic research has shown that the extra fat in overweight and obese individuals interferes with ability of cells to use insulin since fat cells are more resistant to insulin than muscle cells. Another factor believed to contribute is that lipids are stored in skeletal muscle as triglycerides which normally provide fuel for healthy muscles. When the balance between the amount stored and the amount needed for the muscles to perform efficiently is shifted towards excess triglycerides, fat accumulates and obesity develops. Further research in this area is needed to fully understand this physiologic phenomenon.

If you know anyone with diabetes, especially if it is advanced, you know that they worry about or suffer from the complications of diabetes even more so than from the disease itself. One of those complications is end stage kidney disease leading to the need for dialysis. Diabetes is the most common cause of end stage kidney disease. In someone with diabetes, the kidneys can initially compensate for the high blood sugar levels by increasing their ability to filter out the waste products we normally produce. These wastes are excreted in the urine. As they are compensating however, the filtering cells are breaking down and allowing proteins to leak from the blood into the urine. This is called microalbuminuria and is essentially the first sign of damage to the kidneys. Following microalbuminuria, macroalbuminuria develops which means that more albumin and protein is leaking through. Another factor contributing to the breakdown of the kidneys is that an excessive intake of calories puts an overload on the working part of the kidneys leading to impairment. The kidneys ability to filter the blood effectively is altered and waste products build up in the blood stream. These wastes are like poisons and when the levels elevate too much, a person will become symptomatic. Eventually, the kidneys suffer permanent damage and renal failure is present.

Dialysis is a treatment for diabetes that helps to remove the waste products that have accumulated. If you know someone undergoing dialysis, you can probably appreciate how difficult it is. If you are fortunate enough not to know a person who is receiving dialysis, ask a friend or another family member if they know someone. Then ask about their experience and how their life is affected. Learning about the experience of living on dialysis three times a week may be enough to motivate you to avoid this life saving but difficult and demanding situation.

Other consequences of diabetes include blindness from retinopathy (small vessel damage to the eyes), heart attack from damage to small vessels in the heart, and stroke from alterations in the small vessels in the brain. Peripheral neuropathy is another complication of diabetes caused by the injury to small blood vessels in the hands and feet from elevated blood sugar. The main symptom of neuropathy in the earlier stages is pain especially when lying in bed or at rest. There are medications that may help settle down some of the pain but these medications are not effective in all people. When neuropathy becomes more advanced, loss of sensation in the extremities may occur. The concern then is that a wound will develop and go unnoticed until it is severe. With the damage to the small vessels, circulation of blood to the lower legs and feet is impaired making healing more difficult. Diabetic are taught to perform routine inspections of their feet including the bottom and between the toes for early detection and treatment of a problem.

Unfortunately, the most concerning outcome from the combination of these factors is amputation of toes, feet or limbs from wounds which won't heal. Having been a nurse for many years, I have seen the significant impact this has on people. What starts as a few toes requiring amputation may progresses to a foot, a lower leg and eventually an above knee amputation. Unlike traumatic amputation where there is no underlying disease, limb loss from diabetes very often continues to progress. We tragically see people slowly being chipped away. Although there are ways to manage well after an amputation it clearly has a major impact on how one lives.

The thought of developing diabetes should scare us all. What you should know however is that diabetes is preventable by developing good life style habits. And if you already have pre-diabetes, you now know that you can delay or possibly avoid the onset of true diabetes by increasing exercise, losing weight and eating better. Even a diabetic who begins to "get religious" about maintaining a healthier life style can avoid the complications of diabetes. Multiple studies have shown that if people with diabetes maintain good control of their blood sugar, the rate at which complications develop is slowed and even stopped.

Chapter 9

GAIL'S STORY

The reality is that many people cannot change behavior despite knowing it is the right thing for their health. If it were easy, there would not be as much of an industry related to life style changes. Between exercise books, tapes, videos, online programs, diet books and programs, motivational tapes and personal trainers, an enormous amount of money is spent by people trying to get into shape. I would not even have written this book were it not for what I see every day through my work. Recently at a conference focusing on heart disease I listened to lecture after lecture discussing the latest research related to genetics, mechanism of disease, diagnostic tools, procedures, and medications to treat heart disease. Eventually one of the presenters brought up the central point that despite all we know and all the information that is available, none of it matters unless a person is compelled to change behavior. All the research in the world is not going to help unless an individual is willing or able to follow through. Gail is a perfect example of someone who has all the knowledge but is not in the right time or place to make changes. She is the first to admit it.

Gail is a fifty seven year old nurse who works at the same hospital as me. She is like so many women, working full time at a demanding job which requires her to be on her feet most of the day. She also has to be mentally prepared to care for patients with significant physical and emotional needs. She has three grown children and several grandchildren and enjoys spending as much time as possible with her young family.

Perhaps one atypical fact is that Gail has been married to the same man for thirty three years!

Over the past fifteen years or so, Gail has gained about fifty pounds and last summer she was diagnosed with diabetes. In the earlier chapter on diabetes, it was noted that being overweight is a significant contributing factor to the development of diabetes and now unfortunately, Gail has become a statistic. As I was considering who to include for real life stories, it made sense to talk about someone who is struggling with a serious health problem and despite her knowledge is unable to do what she knows is best.

Years ago, as her weight was creeping up, Gail's health care provider told her that the risk of developing diabetes was increasing along with her weight. Despite hearing and understanding this, she thought possibly she would be one of the lucky ones, spared of disease. She also felt that soon she would have time to control her life style and shed some of the extra pounds. Unfortunately, like so many other women, daily life got in the way of accomplishing this goal. Then one day she was given the news that in fact, she was now diabetic and needed to start a fairly common diabetic medication called metformin (Glucophage).

Gail told me that her daily blood sugar checks indicate that the Glucophage is working fairly well although on occasion her sugar runs over 190 which is higher than it should be for good overall control. As we talked further, Gail mentioned that when she exercises, her blood sugar is much better regulated. It was a bit difficult to broach the subject but I did ask her why then would she not just exercise every day or at least most days to help manage her disease. She sighed and tried to answer this question, one she often asked herself.

Throughout the past years, exercise has not been a routine part of her life. At work Gail is busy for hours and by the end of the day, she is worn out. Initially, that was not a big deal but as years crept up, so did the weight. Then menopause hit and the weight gain continued with a vengeance. Gail notes that as time went by, the thought of losing weight became overwhelming. When she tried to drop a bit of weight, it was difficult to stick with a routine. She would exercise and watch what she was eating for a few days or a week, and then something would get in the way of continuing. First it would be a time factor, next time her motivation would wane, next it would be that someone else needed her, then there was the inconvenience of the rain or the snow. Whatever the reason, it was not a matter of knowing what to do; it was mainly an issue of making her wellbeing and exercise a top priority in her life.

When I asked what the major barriers were, she immediately stated that one of the foremost factors is that she always put everyone ahead of herself in regards to needs. Isn't that completely typical of women our age? If it is not the demands of work keeping her there for long hours or the fatigue at the end of the day, it is something she wants to do for her family. The last person on the list of needs is always Gail. She never before had carved out exercise time and now it was exceedingly difficult to change that behavior. Of course, she also admitted that eating more than necessary was part of the problem. The combination of too much food and little or no workout routine had gotten the best of her.

Gail also made a very interesting point regarding the role of her health care provider. She said that discussion about her weight was not part of her routine health care visits. She had received some education about dietary recommendations to better control her cholesterol, but never was the issue of weight loss a specific focus of treatment during her visits. Unfortunately, this is a fairly common finding in part due to the brief time allotted for health care visits but perhaps even more so because weight is a very sensitive issue to chat about. Imagine telling a friend or family member that they are overweight. How you would feel if someone suggested you are too fat? Despite our education, it is difficult for providers to tell someone they are overweight and need to drop some pounds. One never knows how the patient might receive that information.

An interesting medical study a few years ago looked at this issue. People who were overweight were asked whether their provider had covered this topic with them and many said no. They were then asked if they would be bothered if the problem of their weight were brought up and most indicated they would prefer to have an open talk about it. The participants noted that they were not likely to ask about their weight but if the question was openly addressed, they would prefer to discuss it and obtain some advice. In fact, many indicated that having a provider start the discussion may push them to begin to make changes.

The other issues Gail noted as barriers to changing behavior were many of those discussed throughout this book; motivation, commitment, too many other "to dos", not enough time, and on and on She also talked about the impact of denial. Like so many people, Gail had initially figured she would be spared the development of a chronic disease like diabetes. Once she received that diagnosis, her denial changed such that now she holds onto the belief that she will not suffer from the devastating consequences of diabetes which were reviewed previously. When I asked Gail to talk about this denial she said it is not an intellectual thing, it is more an emotional denial. By denying that she will become a victim of her blood sugar, she does not feel badly about not changing her behavior. She can convince herself that it is not a big deal to continue to hold onto her extra weight. Even knowing intellectually that the length of her life may be shortened by living with diabetes is not enough to motivate her, in a significant way due to denial.

So Gail continues to struggle. She makes attempts to get to the gym as often as possible and works on steps to control her diet. She knows that developing an exercise routine would help. She is aware that her family and friends would be supportive of whatever she wanted or needed to do including finding time for herself. She also understands that no one else can make her change; it has to come from within. Still Gail has not found the time in her life to develop a consistent routine. Until she can make changes, Gail said she hopes that her health will not suffer from the consequences of diabetes. She obviously wants to live a long and productive life.

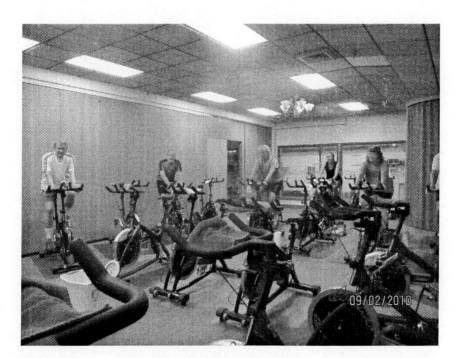

Chapter 10

FIND A FRIEND

One of the greatest incentives to keep you exercising is to make it fun and social. You may wonder how exercise can be fun if you are out of shape and don't necessarily feel like doing it. You need to figure out techniques to put the fun into your exercise.

One way to find joy in exercising is to find a friend to embark on this new adventure with you. Studies have shown that having an exercise companion has a substantial impact on motivation and commitment. There is a bond that develops between exercise partners in the same way that a bond forms in any type of meaningful relationship. Generally neither person wants to break that connection; therefore you are more likely to follow though. The exercise becomes a social event of sorts. As you and your friend begin to become more fit together, the strength of your commitment will blossom. You may have different friends depending on the activity you are doing. Perhaps there is one friend you walk with, a different friend for biking, and someone else to do another activity with, maybe a step aerobics or zumba class.

Recently I started going to spin class at the fitness center where I swim. It was a small group and the attendees mostly knew each other. After several classes I began to catch on to the banter that the participants engaged in particularly between two of the spinners, Jim and Gordon. Jim is a 62 year old retired man who works out at the center almost every day. He has a particular routine which includes spinning several days a week. Gordon attends class several days a week before he heads off to work.

What caught my attention was how their banter helped take the focus off the hard work of the exercise we were doing. Their talk was often about nothing of importance, yet other members of the class would jump into their conversation and the banter would continue for most of the 45 minute class. When either Jim or Gordon is absent, there is a noticeable change in the feeling of the class. Someone will inevitably ask where the boys are and why are they not in class.

Jim also plays tennis one day a week with the spinning instructor and on other days he runs with another club member. Jim said working out with a friend "helps me to get my butt out of bed since I know they are waiting". It is the commitment more so to the other person than to the exercise that is motivation to get going.

Another group who I see most mornings at the center includes several 50ish year old women who meet to work out together. They occasionally start by walking over to Dunkin Donuts to grab a coffee which they drink while they walk in the gym. After their walk, they may go to spin class, Abs with Babs class, swim or any of several other choices. Like many women in their fifties, their weight may not be perfect, but the benefits of ongoing exercise are obvious. I am certain if any of them had to complete a stress test, they would do very well. The important motivator is not just their commitment to fitness but even more so their commitment to each other.

Two of my consistent exercise friends are Michele and Susan. Susan is a fitness fanatic. She is only a few years younger than me but she seems to have a drive that pushes her to excel in whatever activities she undertakes. Susan can leave me in the dust when we exercise together yet because our time together is more than just exercise, she doesn't do that. She slows her pace enough for me to keep up while I am pushing myself harder than usual. Sometimes I think I'm going to collapse. When we work out together we choose an activity that works for both of us where we know I won't slow her down too much. Susan was training for an event that pushed her to work out twice a day, she would do her harder work out in the morning and save her second one to do with me at the end of the day. Sometimes we would choose a run that was easier for me to keep up while she will do a harder run when alone. If Susan wanted to run ahead especially on the hills, she would go for it and come back to meet up with me when I got to the top. Despite our different fitness levels, having the time to talk and catch up was what motivated us to find time and activities that we could enjoy together.

The activity that Susan and I are slightly more compatible at is biking which we would do right from work before going home at the end of the day. When I was riding in the bike portion of the Timberman Short Course Triathlon, I was smiling to myself as I thought about Susan. Since I had been chasing her up hills on my bike throughout the summer, the bike portion of the event seemed easy. Having come out of the swim leg slower than my counter parts, I realized I was passing them on the hills. Thanks to Susan!

Michele is anther friend who I run with mostly in the mornings before work. She is also in her fifties. Michele and I have been running at least once a week for about a year and a half and we run at a more compatible pace. There are days when the last thing I want to do is get up early and start running. It is an especially miserable thought on cold, dark winter mornings. Yet, when the alarm rings I remind myself that Michele will be waiting if I don't show. I also know that at the end of the run I will be happy that I got myself up from my warm bed and set out to meet her. I know that it will be worth the struggle. It is once again that thing of just getting started. Once out there, it is easy to keep going and to love it. Often times after a morning run, one of us will send a quick message during the day to say how great it was to get out.

Having a friend who is slightly more fit that you can provide an additional motivator. On the days you may have to decide whether to get moving and exercise alone, consider how it will help you keep up with your friend. Staying in shape to keep pace may be all you need to prompt you. This is another example of when "mental gymnastics" comes into play. Going through the "should I", "I should because" can be resolved by thinking of working out with your exercise partner.

The best part of having a companion you meet routinely is the friendship that is fostered over time. My runs with Michele give us a chance to catch up on what is going on in our lives and to stay in touch since we don't see each other at work very often. We have both found it to be very therapeutic to share stories and to support each other with whatever issues we are facing. When there is a particularly stressful event or situation to discuss, I often hold onto it until our run. Not only does it help process stressors, having a topic to talk about takes the focus off the muscle burn

One recent day, I was sharing a particularly important moment that had occurred in my personal life. When Michele abruptly stopped and gave me a hug, I realized that she had been living the struggle with me for the previous six months and now she could share in my happiness. Our runs had become so much more than just exercise.

Last winter, Michele and I were planning to meet on a typical cold winter morning. It was still dark, about 22 degrees with a little windy. A really easy morning to skip it. Knowing that she would be waiting, I got myself up and we met at the usual 6:15 time. Often times, we don't have a particular run in mind but have several loops to choose from between 3-6 miles. Although we both had been exercising, neither of us had run in two weeks mostly due to the weather and the holidays. Starting out, I wanted to stick with the 3 mile run but I knew we had a lot of catching up to do. At the one-mile mark were we had to decide on our route, we agreed to the 4 mile run which includes a long hill. Struggling up the hill, I almost regretted our choice until we reached the top. The rest of the run was a sail as we chatted and watched the sun rise. My mind was able to wander away from the hard work to the conversation and the beautiful sky. Later in the day, I received an email from Michele about what a great run it was and what day would work the next week. Her email expressed exactly what I was feeling and although I will face the same challenge to get going on other mornings, I know the run is something I will look forward to.

One approach that can help to keep you committed to your routine and your friend is to make a plan a few days ahead of time. Either the day before or early in the same day, send a text message, email or voice message to your friend early in the day confirming the plan. Rather than asking if the plan is still on, just send a message to firm up the time or meeting place or tell your friend you are looking forward to seeing them. By doing this early, it is more likely that neither person will change their mind and drop out.

I can't finish this chapter without mentioning one other exercise partner, Holly, another 50 something year old friend. When we get together we mostly walk or cross country ski. Often we don't have a particular time frame or route in mind as we head out to the trails in the woods with the dogs. Much of the fun of it is that we just walk and walk and walk exploring trails like kids on an adventure. Generally we know where we are although we have found ourselves almost lost on a few occasions. Of course we talk the entire time barely ever having a pause in the conversation. My time with Holly is more about catching up and sharing in each others lives. The exercise is just the vehicle to find time together.

Any strategy that helps keep you going should be incorporated into your goals. Find little ways that work for you to keep your end of a commitment. The more determined you stay the more your friend will as well.

SO GO OUT AND FIND A FRIEND!!

Chapter 11

MARIA'S STORY

Maria, an almost fifty year old woman, has been married for eighteen years and has a son of eleven. She has been slightly overweight her whole life. In her younger years, Maria actually underwent breast reduction surgery as her size significantly impacted her ability to be involved in physical activities without discomfort. After her surgery, she still never became more active or engaged in athletics on a regular basis.

As Maria grew older she knew it would be beneficial to her health if she started exercising. Throughout her twenties and thirties, Maria tried a number of programs, activities and classes but could not find anything that was captivating enough to keep her going. Early in her forties, she attempted aerobics then spinning class. Neither suited her well so she did not stick with it. Maria, her niece and sister-in-law even joined a yoga class at one point. Her daily job was fairly stressful and not one where she could express her frustration about things that went on. Maria felt that yoga did not fit for her because as she says laughingly "I had an anger issue and could not do it. When everyone else was finding their inner peace, I wanted to hit something". So once again, she quit.

Shortly after that experience, Maria's son was interested in karate so he joined a class at a local martial arts place called Body Works. Once when she was there waiting for him, she saw the advertisement for a kickboxing class. "Now that is something that might work for me" Maria thought and she signed herself up.

Starting an exercise program like kickboxing was a challenge in the beginning. Early on, she could not complete a mere five pushups. Some days she was mentally exhausted and really had to push herself to make it to class. There were days when her body was sore all over. She used several strategies that kept her committed. One thing she did was to pack her gear when she packed her son's so she would have it with her when she dropped him at his class which was right before kickboxing started. By the time he was done, she was mentally ready to jump into her class and she had everything she needed with her so there was no excuse. Maria said she felt the benefits of her exercise early on so rather than thinking about how hard the class would be she reminded herself how good she always felt when done. This worked and she stuck with it and now Maria can do thirty pushups without difficulty. Maria said that incorporating exercise into her life made her feel better about herself not only physically but mentally which helped keep her motivated. Finally she had found an exercise which is perfect for her.

Although Maria has not lost much weight in terms of pounds on the scale, she knows she has lost inches. Her body has become more toned and her clothes fit better. There are times when she is frustrated that the number on the scale has not gone down as much as she would like, yet she knows that inside and outside, she is healthier. Kickboxing gives her a total body work out.

Maria can see the benefits of the exercise in every day things as well. She has made a commitment to using the stairs at work rather than the elevator and can now walk as many flights as needed without feeling winded. Recently, Maria attended an event with some friends and there were no close parking spaces so they had to park a distance away. She noticed that her friends were puffing as they walked along, but she felt completely comfortable with no shortness of breath. Maria had to take the opportunity to teasingly rub it in to her friends noting how much more fit she was now that she was routinely exercising. When she works in her garden or does other chores, she also realizes she can move about so much more easily.

Maria said that she has more energy at the end of the day. She said "I am much less of a slug". Before becoming involved in kickboxing she might not do anything during her evenings. Now she will go out and mow the lawn, take the dog for a walk, do more around the house or go do something active with her son and husband.

It has been two years since Marie joined kickboxing and she is still going to class at least two nights a week and more often when she can. She said she gets a great work out but equally as important, she can release the stress and anxiety that builds during the day. Maria said that when she has had a particularly bad week "I can just kick harder".

A very important point that Maria noted was that the instructor has to be a good fit and at kickboxing she found someone she could bond with. His philosophy of "no competition" except for what you set for yourself was perfect for her. Throughout class, the instructor and the other participants laugh as much as they work out. They might make fun of themselves or each other. She said "Everyone is the same. It is not just a bunch of skinny people looking at me. We are all sweating just as much regardless of how fat or skinny, young or old we are." Maria said once she was feeling particularly fatigued and she told her class that she was too old and fat to be doing this. Not only did everyone laugh but they gave her the extra encouragement she needed to keep going. It is impressive that Maria did not give up. She kept looking for an exercise program that would work for her and after all those years of trying, she has found her place.

Maria is quick to talk about the emotional benefits of exercise. The words she used to describe her experience were; cooperative, supportive, laughter, developing bonds, equal, fun. Even though many of the participants only know each other by first names, they are a cohesive group. When one doesn't come, they all want to know if that person is having any troubles. It is not because of any pressure but they have developed camaraderie. Each member worries about the other when they are absent any amount of time. On those occasions when Maria does not feel like attending, she still goes because "I don't want to let anyone down". She recognizes that this includes herself. She realizes she is always happier when she has been to class.

As with any formal exercise program, there is a cost. For Maria, there have been times when she felt she should stop to save the money. Fortunately her work recognizes the importance of exercise and pays part of the program. Even more fortunate is that her family believes that her routine is important for all of them and have decided her emotional and physical well being is worth the money. If necessary, cut backs will come from somewhere else in the household.

Another factor that Maria recognized as really helpful in keeping her motivated is the example she is setting for her son. She said "I don't want to be a quitter". In the beginning her son may have been a little embarrassed to see his mother out there on the same mat where he did his karate. Over time, she noticed that his feelings about this have changed. Her son and husband have told her how proud they are of her for the progress she has made.

When Maria went through the testing for her blue belt and she passed, her family was there to share in this significant accomplishment. Summed up, Maria says that because of kickboxing "I walk taller".

Chapter 12

EXERCISE STRATEGIES AND GETTTING BEYOND THE EXCUSES

Throughout the previous chapters, numerous strategies to keep you motivated have been suggested. Some of these are repeated here as well as some additional ones listed that don't quite fit the chapter topics. You need to pick which of those will work to keep you committed and to make your routine fun. Also add more to the list as you find the specific tricks that help you.

- Exercising early in the day can be a great way to be sure you do it. One huge advantage is that you don't have to think about it any longer. You are done!! If you go early, it is off your mind leaving you free to think about other the other stuff that is going on.

- When you make your daily "To Do" list, put your exercise on top before the other chores such as pick up laundry, get groceries, wash floor. If you don't have time for all the errands or cleaning, the one thing that is most important to your health will be done. There is always tomorrow to clean the house.

- Find a time when it works to go with family members or a friend and STICK WITH IT. Make it a routine that you don't deviate from. My sister has a friend who she swims with one night a week. They have a preset plan as to who picks up whom, the time they go and how long they are out. They don't deviate from that plan.

- Tell people around you what your plan is so they begin to incorporate that into their routines. Be sure to let them know you need their support to follow through.

- NEVER be the one to pick up that phone to ask your exercise partner if they are still up for going. Use the opposite strategy. If you wonder if they want to go first ask yourself if the real question is do you really want to go? Then go back to your goals and remind yourself of what you are working on. Rather than asking if your buddy wants to go, send a quick message to say you are looking forward to your date.

- If your exercise plan is intermittent with a certain person, contact them early in the day to remind them, as discussed in the chapter on Finding a Friend. If you wait until late in the day, other responsibilities will likely trump your plan. Focusing on your plan can also help you stay on task and complete work so you can be sure to get out on time.

- Join a class where you will see the same group week after week. If you don't know the participants when you start you will get to know them over time. People will expect you to be there and ask you where you were if you miss class.

- Try something new. Think of it as a new adventure. Pick up a zumba class, Pilates or hola hopping. As you begin to learn how to do it your fitness level will be improving which will make it not only fun but easier.

- Develop a group activity. Some of the women at my work started hiking monthly on the night of the full moon utilizing headlamps if needed. As time has gone on, other people (we do allow men to come) have heard of our night hiking group and asked to join in. There is no competition and no reason to hurry along since we are just out there for the fun of being together, doing something different and helping maintain good health in the process.

- Tell someone else (family, friends, coworkers, etc) that you are working on exercising more, losing weight or whatever your main goal is. Keep them updated, within reason of course, on your progress. This also helps motivate you so when they ask how you are doing, you can be proud to share your successes.

- Be careful about rewarding yourself. It is common to hear someone say they exercised and now can eat something gooey and full of calories. Try to reverse this thinking. If you splurge on a delectable food item, tell yourself that now you have to go out and exercise off those calories. Rather than make the food be the reward, make the food be the issue and the exercise be the reward (or punishment depending on your outlook).

- Try the "Five Minute Rule" which is a strategy that deserves its own section and is written about in the next chapter.

Chapter 13

THE FIVE MINUTE RULE

Karen, my sister, is one year older than me. In earlier years, she was one of those people who were up and down on her weight. (Yes, she was upset reading this thinking that I had called her fat!) It was never a huge amount of weight but enough that a new wardrobe was required and she was uncomfortable. She was generally active most of her life but there were lengths of time when activity would go down and a few extra pounds would pack on. I would imagine you know people who "yo yo" on their weight or perhaps you have been one of those.

Karen and her friend Sue used to meet at one of their homes once a week for a run or walk. They would first sit down and chat for a while but as the time slipped away without them heading out the door, the walk or run would not happen. They would do the usual that many of us do of asking "do you really want to go" or "should we go now" or "we really should get going". However, often they would not get going and they would run out of time. Both knew subconsciously that avoidance was the real barrier.

Finally, Sue came up with the Five Minute Rule. She proposed that they start out right away and if after five minutes either of them did not want to keep going, they would return home. After the first five minutes, they would check in to see if either wanted to turn around. Then five minutes later they would check in again. By then they were involved in their walk and would just keep going according to the original plan and time frame.

Getting motivated to start is often the hardest part of an exercise program. Once the body is moving, the endorphins start to kick in, the great feeling of really getting out there takes over and most people want to continue on their journey. For Karen and Sue, this strategy helped to break their habit of avoidance and a new habit of heading out immediately had been created. Karen said that once they implemented the five minute rule they were consistent in following through. It seems like a small step but was huge in changing their behavior and moving towards their goal.

There are a couple other versions of the five minute rule that you can put to use. If you have not been exercising previously, start by only doing five minutes of activity a day or at a time. Think of how many things you might take five minutes to do that could be refocused on exercising. Examples may include having a text conversation, chatting on the phone, picking up after kids, staring out the window thinking about something. If someone asked you to help him or her out doing something like watching their child for five minutes while they ran into the store, or giving them five minutes to do a chore, you would probably not hesitate because it is such a short time.

Tell yourself that every day for the next week you are going to exercise for five minutes. You can march in place, walk up and down the stairs in your house or at work, park far away when doing errands, walk around the grocery store for five minutes before going in or any number of other things. Just commit to five minutes. Then at the end of the week, increase that to ten minutes or two episodes of five minute a day for another week, and then increase from there. Over time, you will learn how to incorporate snippets of exercise time into your busy day. Remember current literature says that 150 minutes of moderate exercise is your goal each week. It is best to spread that out to five days of thirty minutes each day.

Another variation of the five minute rule is one you can use to increase your work out level. If you have been walking as a start, tell yourself that you will increase your pace for five minutes and if you want to back off after that, then go ahead. If you are doing an exercise tape, add weights for just five minutes. Maybe you have decided to join an exercise class. Commit to pushing yourself a little harder for just five minutes during each class. Another avenue would be to arrive five minutes early and warm up, or use a piece of exercise equipment in a gym before starting class. One woman I know runs with her iPod and. when a fast paced tune comes on she increases her speed to keep up with the beat of the song until it is done. This may be for less than 5 minutes but she may use this strategy several times during her run. Over time, your stamina will improve and you will be able to keep pushing yourself using this five minute time frame.

There are certain types of exercise very amenable to the five minute rule. One is exercising your upper body by lifting hand weights. If you don't have any, pick some up today and keep them accessible. Remember muscles burn more calories than fat so building additional muscles will help increase your metabolism. Start slowly with three or five pound weights and do a few repetitions of ten or fifteen lifts each. Do this for five minutes. When you are doing something that allows, like talking on the phone, watching a television program, or having a conversation in the kitchen, grab the weights and knock off a set of lifts. You will be surprised how quickly your muscles will begin to tone. At our age, developing arm muscles gets rid of the triceps skin flap wave and improves our appearance so much.

Abdominal exercises are the other series that fits well into five minutes. Again, vary the type of sit ups choosing from the list below. A group of girls at my daughter's college do a six minute abdominal work out. A mere six minutes a day will build your abs very quickly. Get down on the floor now and do a few sit ups, even if just for 2 minutes. If you have not done those in a while, your abs will be sore tomorrow but that might feel great to you.

Abdominal Exercises
- Do all of these with knees bent
- Put your hands behind your head and lift your upper body up and down as in traditional sit ups
- Lift your torso side to side with your arms out straight moving your arms to the outside of your knees
- Place your hands on the floor next to your butt and lift your legs a few inches off the floor. Hold this position as long as you can
- Place your hands behind your head and brings your knees to elbows on the opposite side while lifting the torso (bicycle sit ups)
- Turn onto your stomach; put your forearms on the floor with elbows at a ninety degree angle. Lift yourself up on your toes and forearms. Hold as long as you can. Try to hold that for

one minute. Your goal is to repeat these three times so work up to that.

So take a five minute break from reading this book right now and do something active. Do abs as above or stand up and just start stretching. Or put your forearms level to your elbows and lift your legs to hit your palms for the next five minutes. You can switch it up and do several things for a minute each. Start with leg lifts as above, then a minute of jumping jacks, sit ups, squats and toe touches. You will feel better even with just five minutes and you will have started your fitness life style. Add "exercise five minutes every day for a week" to your list of goals. GO FOR IT!! YOU CAN DO IT!!

Chapter 14

THE CHALLENGE OF MENOPAUSE

Like it or not, menopause is a part of life that all women need to bear. When you think about your post-menopausal years it is amazing to realize that given our life expectancy, many of us will live almost half our lives in post menopause years!!! When you think about the surge in the number of octogenarians, we can believe this to be a true fact. How one approaches and copes with menopause is very individual.

Regardless of whether we like it or not, the fact is that our bodies will change as a result of menopause and there is nothing we can do to prevent this process from occurring. It is simply the normal physiology of aging taking place. "The Change" however, does not have to be detrimental. Understanding how and why we change will help to manage this transformation.

The literature regarding menopause reveals that the common reactions are to either feel that life is essentially over or to embrace this phase in a way that brings about a new found zest. Some women will welcome menopause and dive in headfirst to take on the challenges without fretting. Some will coast though as just another part of life. Others will dread the onset fearing that this is the beginning of the end of youth. The healthiest is to recognize that these years are a renewed time to make changes and commitments to one's self. Embracing a healthy strategy as one goes through menopause will not only help ease this transition but also provide new opportunities for enjoyment of life. If you focus on the many years ahead, the importance of keeping a strong body becomes obvious. Many women are having children at an older age now, again emphasizing the critical need to stay healthy to see these children become adults as well as to experience the thrill of grandchildren.

The two general stages of menopause affecting women in their 40s and 50s are called peri-menopause and post-menopause. Peri-menopause is the transitional time when the ovaries are starting to change and secretion of the hormones estrogen and progesterone is unpredictable. Peri-menopause may last for several years during which time a woman can expect irregular periods. This is also when you may begin to experience the symptoms related to menopause including hot flashes, disrupted sleeping patterns, forgetfulness, anxiety, weight gain, fatigue, irritability, depression, headache, vaginal dryness, bloating, lack of concentration and many more. Sounds great huh!!

A woman is considered to be post-menopausal when she has not had a period for twelve continuous months. For some women becoming post-menopausal signals a settling down of some symptoms whereas other women will be plagued by signs of estrogen deficiency for years to come. Regardless, of which group you fall into, there are internal body changes taking place that you cannot feel which may be taking a toll. The reason for this is that women are protected to some extent by estrogen. As levels drop off, your body suffers the consequences, some of which may affect you for the rest of your life. Examples of this are deterioration of bones leading to osteoporosis, thinning of the walls of the vagina called vaginal atrophy, increase in cholesterol levels, and slowing down of metabolism. As you go through this stage of life it is critical to realize, to accept and to understand menopause and to decide what you want to do to ease the transition.

There is somewhat limited information available related to how menopause affects weight but there are a couple things to realize as you head into this part of life. Weight gain during menopause is highly likely unless one makes a plan and takes action to prevent weight gain from occurring. This means taking action right away to prevent the weight from going up, even before menopause starts. It is much harder to loose the weight gained once it is there than it is to take steps to prevent it from happening.

When a woman goes through menopause, there is a hormonal alteration in our metabolic rate such that the body requires less energy for normal metabolism. That means the normal physiologic daily activities your body does such as breathe, burn food in the gut, regulate your temperature, respond when you move around, and other internal activities use up less calories to get the job done. Your total basal metabolic rate goes down. The result is that you will gain weight unless you either reduce your intake of calories or you burn calories another way such as by increasing exercise. It simply comes down to when more calories are taken in than what is used weight gain will occur. The supply/demand ratio again. Altering one or the other is essential to maintain a stable weight.

Another physiological fact impacting the equation is that the muscle in our bodies will begin to turn to fat just from the loss of estrogen. Because fat helps with reproduction, women already carry more fat than men. Muscle burns more calories than fat so this switch to having even more fat compounds the imbalance. Fewer calories will be used by the fat which means once again that if you don't figure out how to alter the ratio of calories in versus calories burned, you will gain weight. While it helps to know that it is not your "fault" that you might be getting heavier, you are the only one who can take control and prevent this from happening.

Although we have outlined the negative consequence of weight gain in earlier chapters, there is one additional factor to add to your knowledge. This is especially important since our risk of breast cancer increases as a simple consequence of aging. While the research is not clear, it is believed that for every twenty pounds of weight gain, the risk of breast cancer goes up when compared with women without the weight gain. This is another astonishing fact and one more incentive to avoid packing on the pounds.

Aside from the physiological factors described above, there are a number of psychosocial factors related to menopause that can also contribute to weight gain. Anxiety and/or depression are common during this time of life. This may be particularly true for those women who have been dreading the onset of menopause. But for others, it is more so a consequence of the physical changes from the hormonal fluctuation itself.

One would wonder, why does depression or the blues, start during menopause in women who have not been depressed in the past. Authorities suggest that women experience depression for a number of reasons. The "change" we go through is not only physical, it is emotional. This time is when children are grown up and are leaving or have already left home. Retirement may be just around the corner. We generally take stock of where we have been and where we are going. For some, it is depressing to take an honest look knowing, as mentioned earlier that there are many, many years of life that lie ahead. We may see that we are not really happy with what life has to offer or with where we are. While easier to avoid asking oneself hard questions, as we are faced with the issues than come up in our fifties, it is hard to ignore.

Another factor influencing the menopausal transition is that during this time, many people begin to experience loss of family or friends who have illnesses that become more common with age. For some women, the loss may be a spouse, a significant other or even worse, a child. Loss will not only compound the potential for depression, but may also make it exceedingly difficult to find the motivation needed to keep going. As discussed in the chapters relating Jean and Linda's stories, utilizing exercise as a strategy to cope with the trauma of loss might help get through this time. While post menopause should be and can be a very fulfilling time, often the changes and challenges women experience can be overwhelming.

The daily fluctuations in hormones causing symptoms noted previously can significantly impact how we feel physically. Many women have a more difficult time concentrating and sleep is often interrupted by variations in estrogen and progesterone. Menopause affects sex drive as well as vaginal lubrication, which add to the challenges of feeling amorous. A vicious cycle may start with hormonal changes causing the blues, followed by less energy, and then weight gain occurs. The excess weight leads to fatigue. Lack of sleep adds to the fatigue. Inattention and loss of concentration may be present along with anxiety or the blues. All this leads to further weight gain, we feel less attractive, sex drive lessens..... and now we are traveling further down the spiral.

Think about the younger years when you could eat whatever you wanted and not gain weight. Or before an important occasion, all it took was skipping a meal or lowering food intake for a couple days and any extra weight would come off easily. That tight little black dress would fit the same as always. For most of us, once we hit menopause, those days are gone! Now every pound lost is hard work. Sadly ever pound gained comes on incredibly easily.

You may be wondering, as I did before heading into menopause, if this all really can be true. Are our bodies really that unkind to us? Is it an over exaggeration? Are women really a wreck emotionally or crazy as we have been pegged for so many years? Unfortunately for women, yes it is true that these changes of menopause are real. And no it is not true that you are crazy or embellishing the truth.

I remembering when early in menopause my stomach felt bloated all the time and the waist on all my clothing was tight. The scale also tipped up a few pounds and would not come down. How could that be if I was not eating more? I thought I really must be doing something wrong. Then I went to the play *Menopause the Musical* and it was there that I realized it was not my imagination. Here was a theater full of women (and a few men) laughing about the struggles which we all share. While it was very humorous in the theater, it was a stark reality probably for many of the women sitting there to admit that here we were in that time of life. Some women were like me having had children a little older than some, and faced with teenagers at the same time as starting menopause.

This book will not discuss hormone replacement therapy (HRT) as it is a very lengthy subject that continues to be somewhat controversial. HRT is a personal decision and one is beyond the scope of this book. I can tell you that I utilize hormone replacement to help manage my symptoms, the worst for me being the sleeplessness. While hormone replacement controls the signs of menopause, it does not help with the bloating and the weight gain, especially around the waist. So back to the exercise and calorie intake issues. For those interested in HRT, additional information can be found on this topic of course on the internet, in books or through a health care provider

If weight gain is a result of the change in metabolism discussed above, there are really only two choices; either eat less or exercise more. The magnitude of one or the other does not have to be huge, just enough to reestablish a balance. The amount of calories you need to focus on is only 200-400 per day. That means either eating 200-400 less calories or burning that many more or a combination of the two. While that might seem like a lot, there are many little things that can have a big impact. It is all the very little things that can add up easily to that many calories. The little taste of something, the one snack you grab when stopping for gas, or the addition of one extra piece of cheese to an item all will have a bang on the bottom line.

Chapter 17 discusses diets and tips related to food choices. The list below includes a few other tips so pick out additional steps that you feel you might be able to implement to address the calorie imbalance. Just these simple steps can eat up those extra calories.

- Curb the temptation to pick. A little extra bite here and there adds calories very quickly.

- When you can't avoid picking, choose something low calorie like carrots or fruit rather than high calorie items like potato chips.

- Pick a lower calorie version of something you like. Consider yogurt as an example. There are so many varieties available. Take the time to look at the labels. Vanilla yogurt in one variety might have 150 calories a cup where another will have only 80. Dannon Light and Fit is my favorite. With only one third of the calories of some other brands this alone affects those 200 calories you are trying to spare!

- Avoid the little dishes of hard candy. Each little piece can have as much as 50 calories. Other "penny candy" carries similar calories.

- Never go through the "drive thru" window for the bank, your coffee, your prescriptions or anything else. Parking and walking in can burn several calories.

- Park a bit further away when you do go into a store. The extra walk will help.

- Always take the stairs rather than the elevator. THAT MEANS BOTH UP AND DOWN. At first it will seem like a lot of work but this is a great way to get a little exercise throughout your day and over time it will get easier. At work, when I take the stairs I play a little game and try to beat the elevator riders up. People will be impressed when they get off and see that you got there faster and are already walking down the corridor.

- Walk as much as you can throughout your day. Take a few extra trips to the bathroom, the water fountain, to do an errand at work. If you are at home, take a few purposeful extra trips up and down the stairs.

- When you feel ready, try to progress to brisk walking or slowly jogging a little from one place to another. Try that instead of walking even if only for a brief stint.

- Get some hand weights for home and use them for a few minutes whenever the time is available. As mentioned earlier, our muscle mass goes down during menopause. Muscle toning helps utilize calories better as well as help to burn more calories with normal activities.

• When you can, stand rather than sit. A new study was conducted on the benefits of standing. A very surprising finding was that standing even in one place without much movement utilizes a significantly higher amount of calories than sitting. Do this when you go to a sporting even, a lecture or any other possible place. If someone asks why you are standing and you don't want to tell the truth, just tell them you have a back issue and it is more comfortable.

The bottom line is that the only way to avoid the fateful consequence of menopause is to take control immediately. You can transition through this time with ease. Utilizing the steps outlined throughout this and other chapters will certainly help. Have no doubt, however, that doing nothing will lead to physical changes you may not like. Exercise is essential as it can facilitate the transition and lessen many of the problems faced during this life-altering phase.

Chapter 15

JEANNE AND LINDA'S STORIES

Jeanne was 54 years old when her husband John passed away after a long term illness. Jeanne had cared for John for many years, providing total care in the last six months of his life. Two years earlier, Jeanne had also lost her son, unexpectedly and tragically. Although she had grieved, her attention was quickly diverted to John's declining physical situation. Living in the long winters of Maine in a somewhat isolated town, she had to do everything from stacking all the wood to complete maintenance of their home and yard to making all the decisions.

Before John was completely unable to move about, Jeanne packed up and moved to Southern California where she had family close by and the weather was more cooperative. Jeanne joined a fitness center soon after her move however; as time went on she could only get away when another family member was able to be at home with John. Still Jeanne knew that she had to take advantage of these opportunities to exercise even a little bit because this not only helped her to feel physically better, it also gave her emotional strength beyond what she innately had. Jeanne found occasions when she was able to get out for a walk with her sister and a few of the women she had come to know. As challenging as it was to get out, she went as often as she could realizing that both the exercise and the socialization was critical to supporting her otherwise difficult life

After John died, one of Jeanne's most important routines was to continue her activities. Given that she did not have any specific responsibilities at home, Jeanne went to the fitness center every day. She said it was the "glue that held her together" as she established a new routine and learned to live life alone. She described the other benefits this way

"going to work out was a way I could be with other people but it was on my terms. I did not always want to get together with friends and family because it forced me to make plans ahead of time as well as to work around their schedule. At that point, I was getting through one day at a time and often found it difficult to mentally plan ahead. Well meaning friends wanted me to talk about how I was doing and the next steps in my life but at times I did not want to or could not talk or think about that.

At the gym, I could talk to people if I wanted but it did not have to be about anything except superficial stuff. That is what I needed. When I was exercising, my mind could go some place else where I did not have to think about anything stressful. I could just be there doing my thing with other people but not really having to interact.

After working all day and then being at the gym, I would go home tired enough that I just had something to eat and then went to bed. There was less time to feel lonely in my home. I was not trying to escape but this helped me to begin the difficult transition to a new life without John."

There were other times when Jeanne would need to or want to talk about her struggles. Then she would go on walks with Karen and other friends as she had when John was alive. Jeanne talked about the turmoil of the previous several years. There were no easy answers, only questions to be processed. Walking and talking provided an outlet to help her cope with her significant losses.

Never can it be said that this was an easy time for Jeanne, but according to her, the exercise and the friendships helps to ease the pain to some degree. How much the endorphins helped will never be known, but the "runner's high" at least can provide moments of feeling better. Eventually the better moments begin to be more frequent than the terrible moments and now four years later, Jeanne is finding her way.

LINDA'S STORY

Linda's is another story of how exercise provided an outlet through a difficult time in life. Her story also speaks to the value of having friends to plan activities with on a routine basis.

Linda is a fifty four year old woman who lives in California and works as manager of an insurance firm. At twenty, Linda fell and broke her pelvis, left knee and upper leg bone, the femur. She had a surgical plate put in but some time later developed an infection. The plate had to be taken out and once recovered, she started physical therapy.

Linda had been someone who was active off and on but was about 20 pounds overweight. She felt physical therapy was boring and knew that she should be exercising more but was just not doing so. She and a friend started going to a program for women called Gym and Swim. At first, as with starting any new exercise activity, the swimming was challenging. She said "I almost gave up it was so hard". She started slowly swimming the side stroke, then incorporated new strokes, all the time increased her distance. Eventually Linda was able to build up to a full mile. Then busy life got in the way and she cut back on her exercise.

When Linda hit her thirties, she had put on some weight and decided it was time to start exercising again because she said it was "important for my head". She realized that taking walks and hikes was the easiest activity to incorporate into her schedule. She had five or so friends who were often available to go out with her so she developed some routine walks that she could look forward to. . Linda continued intermittently with a variety of activities from then but never did she realize that all too soon, exercise would become more essential than just for her physical well being.

When Linda was fifty-one, her husband died from cancer. During the time before he died, she had been consumed with taking care of him and staying by his side. Many months after his death, she began to dig herself out of the hole left in her. Not only was she an emotional wreck, she remembers feeling terrible about how her body felt. Linda described the feeling as "slothful". It was at that time she resumed her exercise in part because of her physical state but also because she realized that this was a way to begin healing emotionally. Getting back to an exercise routine was one way to help her deal with her huge loss.

As also mentioned in Jeanne's story, Linda would exercise after work so she could come home tired and just go to sleep. The workouts helped fill up her time thereby avoiding the loneliness. During that time, she started swimming again. Her first swim was challenging to the point where she did not know if she would be able to do it. Linda stuck with it and slowly over time, her strength and stamina grew. Now she swims as often as possible. One of the benefits of swimming is as Linda notes, there is a peacefulness that is hard to find with other activities. Early on, it was a way for her to get into her head and grieve without having to share her thoughts. It provided her an avenue to process the significance of her marriage, the passing of her husband, her place in life and the future ahead. Another benefit was that arthritis was threatening her knees from her previous injury. Pounding activities were difficult and left her in pain when she was done, but at the same time, Linda knew that exercise was essential to manage her arthritis. Swimming was the perfect activity for so many reasons and one that she continues to do today.

When talking about what keeps her motivated, Linda said that now routine exercise is critical for her in part because of the good physical feeling the exercise brings but also for the pride she feels in herself. Linda said that "I can do it and good for me". If she misses a few days, her mental energy declines allowing unhappy feelings to set in and the sloth to return. Linda admits she also has a slightly competitive side that helps push her when she is engaged in activities with others. When working out with other women she does not want to let them burn more calories than her so she works harder. If someone is moving faster up the hill than her, she will pick up her pace. Her competitiveness does not interfere and may not even be noticeable to her exercise companion, more so, it helps her achieve her personal goals. Linda recognizes also the fellowship that builds when having an exercise partner to join on a routine basis. She values her private swimming time as much as her shared time with friends.

Perhaps the most important thing Linda mentioned is the awareness that at the end of the day her body and her mind feel better for having exercised. It is this good feeling that she relies on to get her going the next day. Not only did her routines carry her through a tragic and trying time but now as she continues to heal, her routines help reinforce that life can go on despite tragedy and that "life is good". She stated that exercise is "the one thing that I can always do just for myself".

Chapter 16

IDEAL BODY WEIGHT

Exercise alone is one strategy to improve health and fitness and to loose weight. Coupled with dieting, weight loss will likely occur more quickly and the benefits will be compounded. In fact, some experts suggest that while exercise will definitely improve health, lower blood pressure and cholesterol levels, and advance diabetes control, without adding a diet regime to that, the results will be slower.

If weight loss is your goal, it is important to really buy into the belief that muscle is heavier than fat. You may know this intellectually yet find it difficult to believe when you are working really hard and not seeing the results on the scale. Your body may be changing and your clothing may fit better even though you may not actually see as much change on the scale as you hope or expect.

For some, it may be best to avoid checking your weight so you won't be discouraged. Others can't resist checking the scale. If you are one of those, be sure to include other measurements as well such as waist size or clothing size. Also, keep a close eye on other health parameters such as blood pressure, cholesterol levels or blood sugar as you get fit. Use the lowering of those numbers as a positive reinforcement that your workouts are paying off. It may help you to keep a chart of your physical activity each day so you can see how much more you can do as the days go on.

If you watch the weight loss shows or competitions on television, it is easy to be impressed with contestants who can loose 10 or more pounds in a week. You may wonder why you can't loose that much weight as quickly. As time goes by, the same contestant will see the weekly weight loss decrease. Additionally, the people who start out lighter have a much more difficult time loosing as much weight over the same time period. Realize that when a very obese person initially starts a weight loss program, the weight will come off fairly easily because they have so much to lose. As the weight drops, their overall percentage of fat is less and the loss slows down. These individuals are also exercising and building more muscle. As we noted earlier muscle weighs more than fat contributing even further to the slowing of weight loss.

Have you ever heard someone say they lost weight but they can't shed the final five or ten pounds? It is in part due to this same physiology and realize that the same will be true for you no matter how much you weigh. Set you goals accordingly.

So how much should you weigh? The best resource to help you decide that is a body mass index (BMI) chart, a well-established tool to use as a guide for what your weight should be for your height. This will determine if you are the ideal weight, underweight, overweight, or obese. It can help you to develop your weight goals. The NHLBI also has a link to a web site that will simply calculate the BMI for you. The limitations of the BMI are noted on their link but realize that it is not a perfect tool. There can be an overestimation of BMI in individuals such as athletes who are muscular and an underestimation in people who have lost body muscle mass. Work towards getting the weight into the normal or ideal body weight category.

A friend was sharing a story related to the weight and BMI. She had never owned a scale until her husband brought an extra one home from work. Her daughter, who was 17 years old, started weighing herself and found that she weighed more than she thought. She is an active, healthy, athletic, beautiful girl who now was obsessed with the numbers on the scale rather than on how she looked and felt. She was working out a lot for soccer and had a significant degree of muscle mass. At her age, it was devastating for her to see those numbers but when her Nurse Practitioner calculated her body mass index, she was exactly where she should be: not too heavy and not too thin. So they put the scale away and she continued to focus on what she was eating and how much she was exercising. She rarely rechecks her weight now because the numbers were too overwhelming and depressing. As long as her clothing fits, she knows she is not gaining weight.

On the other hand, for some people, watching the numbers fall on the scale helps to stay motivated and in that case, one should certainly check their weight. It may be better not to check every day because there definitely will be fluctuations up and down. Focus on the goal of a certain number of pounds over a certain period of time. But again remember that muscle weighs more than fat so the scale may not go down as much as you feel it should. At the same time if you are dropping clothing sizes or your clothes are fitting differently, trust that your body is changing regardless of what you see on the scale.

There are some health conditions where checking a daily weight on a scale regularly is necessary. Some people with heart disease, specifically heart failure, need to check their weight every day since this can be a sign of fluid retention. Also, if you are diabetic, keeping tabs on weight loss is important since this could impact medications taken to control diabetes, especially insulin. As a diabetic looses weight, glucose is better controlled and routine medications may need to be lowered.

As we talked about earlier, don't forget that as women age it is more difficult to loose weight and maintain that weight loss because of how our body metabolism changes. So while normal weight is the goal, if you start exercising and loose some weight, your overall health will improve and you can add years to your life. Unlike when we were younger and wanted to be a certain weight, as we age our target can change. There are people who have a few extra pounds but are still healthy based on how they live and the choices they make. Staying active is probably more important as we age than keeping a perfect weight.

Go back to the goals you set if you are ever discouraged by your progress. Consider if you have met any of your goals. If you are not loosing as much weight as you want but you have increased your activity for example, be proud. If your BMI is improving, know that you are making progress. If you have gotten out the door to exercise close to as many times as you wanted to, be happy. Weight loss is a very slow process and weight that comes off slowly along with lifestyle changes is likely to stay off. Weight that comes off quickly with special diets is more likely to go back on because life style changes have not become well established. Better health through fitness and dietary improvements has to become a way of life rather than a short term experience.

Body Mass Index Table

	Normal						Overweight					Obese									Extreme Obesity															
BMI	19	20	21	22	23	24	25	26	27	28	29	30	31	32	33	34	35	36	37	38	39	40	41	42	43	44	45	46	47	48	49	50	51	52	53	54
Height (inches)											Body Weight (pounds)																									
58	91	96	100	105	110	115	119	124	129	134	138	143	148	153	158	162	167	172	177	181	186	191	196	201	205	210	215	220	224	229	234	239	244	248	253	258
59	94	99	104	109	114	119	124	128	133	138	143	148	153	158	163	168	173	178	183	188	193	198	203	208	212	217	222	227	232	237	242	247	252	257	262	267
60	97	102	107	112	118	123	128	133	138	143	148	153	158	163	168	174	179	184	189	194	199	204	209	215	220	225	230	235	240	245	250	255	261	266	271	276
61	100	106	111	116	122	127	132	137	143	148	153	158	164	169	174	180	185	190	195	201	206	211	217	222	227	232	238	243	248	254	259	264	269	275	280	285
62	104	109	115	120	126	131	136	142	147	153	158	164	169	175	180	186	191	196	202	207	213	218	224	229	235	240	246	251	256	262	267	273	278	284	289	295
63	107	113	118	124	130	135	141	146	152	158	163	169	175	180	186	191	197	203	208	214	220	225	231	237	242	248	254	259	265	270	278	282	287	293	299	304
64	110	116	122	128	134	140	145	151	157	163	169	174	180	186	192	197	204	209	215	221	227	232	238	244	250	256	262	267	273	279	285	291	296	302	308	314
65	114	120	126	132	138	144	150	156	162	168	174	180	186	192	198	204	210	216	222	228	234	240	246	252	258	264	270	276	282	288	294	300	306	312	318	324
66	118	124	130	136	142	148	155	161	167	173	179	186	192	198	204	210	216	223	229	235	241	247	253	260	266	272	278	284	291	297	303	309	315	322	328	334
67	121	127	134	140	146	153	159	166	172	178	185	191	198	204	211	217	223	230	236	242	249	255	261	268	274	280	287	293	299	306	312	319	325	331	338	344
68	125	131	138	144	151	158	164	171	177	184	190	197	203	210	216	223	230	236	243	249	256	262	269	276	282	289	295	302	308	315	322	328	335	341	348	354
69	128	135	142	149	155	162	169	176	182	189	196	203	209	216	223	230	236	243	250	257	263	270	277	284	291	297	304	311	318	324	331	338	345	351	358	365
70	132	139	146	153	160	167	174	181	188	195	202	209	216	222	229	236	243	250	257	264	271	278	285	292	299	306	313	320	327	334	341	348	355	362	369	376
71	136	143	150	157	165	172	179	186	193	200	208	215	222	229	236	243	250	257	265	272	279	286	293	301	308	315	322	329	338	343	351	358	365	372	379	386
72	140	147	154	162	169	177	184	191	199	206	213	221	228	235	242	250	258	265	272	279	287	294	302	309	316	324	331	338	346	353	361	368	375	383	390	397
73	144	151	159	166	174	182	189	197	204	212	219	227	235	242	250	257	265	272	280	288	295	302	310	318	325	333	340	348	355	363	371	378	386	393	401	408
74	148	155	163	171	179	186	194	202	210	218	225	233	241	249	256	264	272	280	287	295	303	311	319	326	334	342	350	358	365	373	381	389	396	404	412	420
75	152	160	168	176	184	192	200	208	216	224	232	240	248	256	264	272	279	287	295	303	311	319	327	335	343	351	359	367	375	383	391	399	407	415	423	431
76	156	164	172	180	189	197	205	213	221	230	238	246	254	263	271	279	287	295	304	312	320	328	336	344	353	361	369	377	385	394	402	410	418	426	436	443

Chapter 17

WHICH DIET IS BEST?

A book about health, exercise or fitness would not be complete without a section on dieting. So, when starting to write this chapter, I did an online search using the heading "Diets". The initial list that came up included 74 diets and it was not an exhaustive list as there were some I knew about that were not included!! Most diets have a theme of course from avoiding carbohydrates, to lowering fats, to supplemental shakes, to eating only fruits and vegetables, to cabbage soups or cleansing remedies. How then do you decide which diet is the best? Which diet is the most effective?

Someone said to me once that if any of these diets worked then why is there a multibillion-dollar diet industry in our country. That really made sense because the bottom line is that none of these diets work if you don't stick to it and all diets will work if you eat less calories than what you are burning. What that means is that you don't need a book or any of the diets or foods supplied by a dietary company if you just do what the generations before us did which is to eat smart, avoid over eating and stay active.

Ask yourself right now: What is the right way to eat? I feel certain that you know much of the answer. Perhaps it would help for you to have a bit more education about specific factors, yet overall you know the basic rules of what to eat:

- lots of fruits and vegetables
- less foods that are high in fat, especially saturated fats and trans fats

- little or no foods high is refined sugars (white sugar, corn syrup)
- fresh foods rather than processed foods
- little or no "junk foods"
- more whole grains than refined grains
- lean meats
- fish and chicken which are high in protein and low in fat if the skin is removed
- low calorie food rather than high calorie food
- limit eating out in restaurants at least initially
- vitamins and minerals at the recommended daily requirements
- sufficient intake of calcium, especially for women
- it is OK to eat something that is "bad for you" on occasion as long as it is in moderation
- alcohol in limited amounts is not harmful but does add calories
- and yes, it is true, that you should avoid ALL fast food restaurants unless you have carefully reviewed the contents and calories of the item you are choosing

So if you know what to do, what is the problem? Probably the biggest barrier in making dietary changes is breaking habits. Changing your diet means shopping differently, cooking differently and of course eating differently. Initially, it will take more time to shop and cook but it will get easier as you learn about new foods and new recipes. The investment in that time is so incredibly valuable as you will see once you get beyond the initial steps and incorporate the changes into your life.

An equally significant barrier may be the people around who you cook for or who eat with you both at work and at home. Share your goals and objectives so they understand why you are making changes. Ask them for their support and remind others that they will benefit as well if they care to make changes. If the important people in your life don't want to make changes, don't put any pressure on them to change. Ask for their help by giving you support and avoiding putting any pressure on you. Change is challenging for everyone and takes time to accept. Expect that your family members may find your dietary changes difficult to deal with however, by eliciting their support, everyone will benefit.

As an example of how change can take time and persistence, I think of my husband and his work colleagues and their daily routine. His office group would order out for lunch every day from any number of local restaurants. With two children in college and his need to drop some weight, he decided that packing lunch was one change he could make so he started to do that most every day. Initially it was not only a big change for him but also for his co-workers. There had been a sort of daily ritual of deciding where to order lunch, collecting money and eating together. Both he and his co-workers felt like he was no longer part of the group. He previously had often volunteered to pick up the meals so others had to step forward and take over that task. Now that time has gone by, he is eating less, making better food and calorie choices, and definitely not spending as much money. His peers have also become accepting of this change and a new routine has been established. One immeasurable step that helped him to change habits was that when making dinner at night, we either make lunches for the next day or make enough extra for leftovers. Then there is no excuse to buy lunch out from a restaurant.

When considering your diet, the first step is to figure out your daily calorie needs based on your size and activity level. There are many available online resources where you can plug in your data and your recommended caloric intake will be calculated. (Try www.freedieting.com/tools/calorie_ calculator) Or you can figure this our on your own using these steps:

1. Know your desirable weight range for your height from the BMI chart.
2. Multiple that by 10.
3. Determine your activity level. Multiply that by your weight. If sedentary, multiply your weight x 3, if moderately active x 5 and if strenuously active x 10.

Example: If your desirable weight is 120 pounds then 120 X 10 =1200. If you are moderately active, then 120 X 5 = 600. Add 1200 + 600. Your daily caloric needs equal 1800 calories to maintain your current weight. To loose weight, calorie intake will need to be lower.

It is very common to think that you are eating fewer calories than you actually are so establishing a baseline is crucial. Before you embark on dietary changes, look at how many calories you are eating in a day. Keep track of your intake for a few days, then figure out your current total caloric intake. Be sure to include EVERYTHING you eat, even those small bites of food here and there that you think don't really count. One advantage of understanding your daily intake is that you might discover easy steps you can take to drop the calories. As noted earlier, just substituting something like carrot sticks or an apple for crackers or the granola bar you have at break can make a big difference.

The next important step in adapting to a new diet is to read food labels and keep track of your intake of fats for a period of time. You can do this along with tracking your caloric intake or tackle one issue at a time. One of the reasons the diet programs that sell food or meals are successful is that they do all this work for their customers. Rather than having to figure out how much of what it is that you consume, all you have to do is purchase their products and eat according to their plan. There are many down sides to that beyond the money that is spent such as what to do if you are eating at someone else's house, or when you go to a party, or are out longer than you planned and pre-purchased food is not available.

A word of caution is needed here as you try to change your diet by reading food labels. You must pay attention to what the serving size is, figure out how much you are eating in terms of number of servings then calculate the total intake from there. For example a can of soup probably has 2 ½ servings in the can. There may be 800mg of salt and 7 grams of total fat with 1.5 gram of saturated fat per serving. That can of soup may not be terribly large or filling so you may eat half or all of what you cook. You then need to do the math to accurately figure out your intake. If you eat the whole can, you would have eaten 2000 mg of salt, 17-18 grams of fat, and 4.5 grams of saturated fat. Depending on your daily calorie needs, that may be half of the daily recommended amount of fat. For someone with heart disease or high blood pressure and on a sodium restricted diet, much of the recommended salt would be consumed in one meal. Add a sandwich and some chips to your meal and you may be at or over your recommended maximum for the day. Replace that meal with something like a healthy half sandwich on whole grain bread and cauliflower cheese soup made with skim milk and low fat cheese and you can fill up and still be far below your limit.

Perhaps the most important reason not to follow one of these diets is that you never learn how to control the diet yourself. At some time in the future, you will want to go off the plan that you are paying for and then what do you do. It makes sense to know how to read food labels and to keep track of your intake. In my experience, many consumers are often very surprised when they really take a look at the contents of certain foods that they have always considered to be somewhat healthy. Start by educating yourself.

Lowering the fat, especially saturated fats is especially important to cut calories but also to reduce the risk of plaque build up as discussed in Saving Your Heart chapter. To start, you need to figure out if you are eating too much fat and how to decrease that amount. Fats contain 9 calories per gram while other foods like proteins contain 4 calories per gram. The recommended intake of fats in the average diet is less than 30% of the total calories eaten. Some experts even suggest lowering the fat intake to 20% of daily calories That means if you eat 1500 calories a day, less than 300 (20%) to 450 (30%) of those calories should come from fats. That can be translated into grams of fat per day by dividing the calories by 9 calories per gram. Use the chart below to determine your recommended grams of fat.

MAXIMUM RECOMMENDED GRAMS OF FAT PER DAY

Daily Calories	Fat Calories	20% of Calories	30% of Calories
1200	240-360	27	40
1400	280-420	31	47
1500	300-450	33	50
1600	320-480	36	53
1700	340-510	38	56
1800	360-540	40	60
2000	400-600	44	67
2200	440-660	49	73
2400	480-720	53	80
2600	520-780	62	93

There are different types of fats, some which are bad for us and contribute to blockage from plaque buildup in our arteries and some which are not harmful. Saturated fats and trans fats are the type of fat that should be limited or avoided as much as possible. Monounsaturated and polyunsaturated fats are essential to include in our daily diet as long as these are in moderation. The general guideline for the breakdown of the fats is that no more than 10% from saturated fats, no more than 10% from polyunsaturated fats and the rest from monounsaturated fats.

It may be confusing and seem like a lot of work to figure this all out but it is really not that difficult if you take it a little at a time. Once you learn the right foods, these will become part of your routine and shopping will be very easy. Just like with exercise, take it a little at a time. Choose a common product you purchase and when you are in the store, pick up a couple other brands and compare the labels for the essential ingredients. Perhaps try the one lowest in calories and fats. If you don't particularly like it try another brand next time.

Recently when shopping I saw an older couple who were walking up and down the isles comparing labels together. They each had a brand and were reading aloud each line item. After comparing several choices, they would decide which to put into the cart. They were clearly making informed purchases. Many major grocery stores now have programs to help you shop better. Some will offer events such as shopping with a dietician. Some have certain labeling throughout the store for healthier foods. Check at your store for programs such as these. Another great resource is your local hospital which may provide educational lectures on nutrition and diet.

If all the work of reading labels, figuring out your intake, comparing foods and cooking new recipes is too much for you right now, there are some basic changes you can make immediately that assure you are lowering calories and fats. Basic principles would include:

- Purchase dairy products that are low fat or fat free including changing to skim milk. Here is a health tip for your future generations. If you have children or grandchildren, start now to transition them to skim milk by doing a half skim/half whatever they now drink. Once they are used to that, lower to two thirds skim/one third other, then three quarters/one quarter and finally just skim milk. Eventually 2% or whole milk will not taste good. This is especially important for teenage boys who tend to drink gallons of milk.

- If you eat yogurt, check the fat content and calories. These vary substantially between products. If you don't eat yogurt, give it a try. This is a great food to add to your diet. Dannon Light and Fit is delicious, low fat and only 80 calories. It also contains calcium.

- Don't use butter or margarine in anything that you can

substitute a good oil like olive oil. Try this with different recipes. If you can't substitute completely use ½ oil and ½ the butter or margarine.

- Get rid of dessert foods like cookies, candies, ice cream, or anything with a frosting such as in breakfast items. Eat foods like this very infrequently and in moderation.

- Avoid all chips and snack foods unless you read the label and you are sure it is low in saturated fats.

- Carry healthy snacks with you all the time. You will be less likely to run into the corner store and grab something unhealthy. A bag of baby carrots is a great item to bring along each day. Or pack a few pieces of fruit for those hungry moments.

- Crunchy foods like carrots and pretzels will fill you up while also satisfying the need to eat. They also tire the jaw out so you may get tired of chewing.

- Eat more fish and chicken breast. Take the skin off before cooking.

- Avoid snacking between meals as much as possible.

- Eat less meat. If you are eating meat, choose lean types. Ask the butcher for help.

- Freshly cooked foods almost always will contain less fat, calories and salt than prepackaged foods.

- Choose whole grain breads, pasta, rice and other such items.

Another area where you may be getting more calories and fat than you think is in the restaurant. When you eat out, despite ordering fairly healthy food, there generally will be more quantity than you need and therefore more calories. When you don't prepare the food, you also don't know what has been added that raises the total calories. For example, did you ever wonder why the steamed broccoli or other vegetables in restaurants is so delicious? It is because butter is added when these are cooked and possibly in a higher quantity than what you would put on at home. You can ask for the vegetables without butter in most restaurants. The sauces on foods in restaurants are usually very high in calories and fats so choose wisely. A wine sauce or red sauce will be better than a cream, butter or cheesy sauce. Another tip is to order a salad with dressing on the side. This will fill you up some before you meal. Then bring home the left overs to have later.

Eating out occasionally is fine even when on a diet, as long as you pay attention to the balance. Planning ahead of time for your night out will help immensely. The Heart Wellness Program at my hospital which is for people with heart failure teaches them how to cheat. We have county fairs several times a year which most local people like to attend. The sausage sandwiches and many other delectable choices there can really get someone in trouble. So we recommend really cutting back the few days beforehand and afterward to allow for the sinful foods that everyone loves. This is a strategy that can work for you as well. The mistake is when you cheat all the time. This should only be an occasional event.

Perhaps the most challenging problem in all this is not which diet is best for you but rather how do you stay motivated and stick to a diet. Figuring out the answer to this question is the only way for you to get on and stay on the dieting path. Start by educating yourself about healthy foods and dietary behaviors then little by little incorporate changes into your diet. You may want to start out by making modifications gradually or it might work better for you to go cold turkey. Perhaps you can clear out all the unhealthy foods from your cabinets and take them to a food kitchen. Unfortunately food kitchens don't have as much choice about what to feed people and will be happy to take your nonperishable items. Go back to your goals and objectives as often as you need to. Post signs to reminder yourself and the people around you of your goals.

One strategy that you can try is to plan when you are going to splurge and have something you really like. This will prevent the guilt or the feeling that you lack will power. If the item is not a desert, have that along with a lower calorie item like a salad or fruit. If it is a luscious desert item rather than having a meal and then having desert, just eat that item as your meal. Another trick that works is to postpone the day of the splurge if you can. This does take away some spontaneity but is just like planning ahead for anything. Pick a day that you will allow yourself to have a treat. When that day comes around, try to put it off another day. Then the next day, see if you can wait another day. This really works and gets back to the notion of not looking too far ahead in regards to goals. We all know that like little children, when we can't have something we want it even more. Setting a goal of avoiding your favorite treat for two weeks is more difficult than looking only a couple days ahead and delaying another couple days when the time comes. If you cannot stand to put it off another day or two, just go ahead and give in. Then wait another period of time before doing it again. All of this erases the self guilt and disappointment with not following a diet. The other trick that can work especially at home is to use a smaller serving bowl that you normally would. Your portions will be better controlled.

One last suggestion that a patient actually told me is to "MAKE HUNGER YOUR FRIEND". A huge part of why we eat of course is because we feel hungry. For most of us however, if we don't eat for another hour or two, we will be fine. So get used to the feeling of hunger. This helps the stomach size to shrink which will eventually help you to feel less hungry. The mid section of your body will feel thinner when you are hungry which will reinforce that you are loosing some weight or at least some body size. I am not suggesting that you skip meals but becoming comfortable with being a little bit hungry will help you to put off snacking until you can sit down and eat something nutritious, healthy and low calorie. Acknowledging the feeling of hunger also prevents between meal snacking which will lower daily calories substantially. Just to reinforce a point here though, if you can't hold off on snacking for whatever reason, choose something crunchy and healthy.

One final step to consider is when you eat a meal stop eating before you feel full. I am sure you have heard this many times before but it really does work. Inevitably, most people eat at least a little more than they need in order to fill up but the fullness does not usually catch up until after the meal is over. If you stop a bit sooner, you will feel full with less food. Over time, this again help the stomach to shrink and the hunger feeling to be more controlled. One strategy in an earlier chapter is worth mentioning again. At the end of the meal, go for a walk. It may help you to eat less and will help to digest the food. Perhaps put this on your list of goals.

There are two diets in the literature that incorporate many useful points and that you don't have to spend any extra money to follow. These are the Mediterranean Diet and the DASH Diet which was developed by the Federal Government. Each of these has been extensively utilized in many clinical research trials and is well accepted as improving heart health. These diets include some additional points beyond those listed above. For example, the DASH Diet as mentioned in the chapter on Blood Pressure suggests lowering the salt in the diet. The Mediterranean Diet suggests that adding olive oil and lots of grains in the diet is beneficial. Details about both of these diets are available online at http://www.nhlbi.nih.gov/health/public/heart/hbp/dash for the DASH diet and http://www.mayoclinic.com/health/mediterranean-diet for the Mediterranean Diet. An internet search will of course list additional resources for each of these diets.

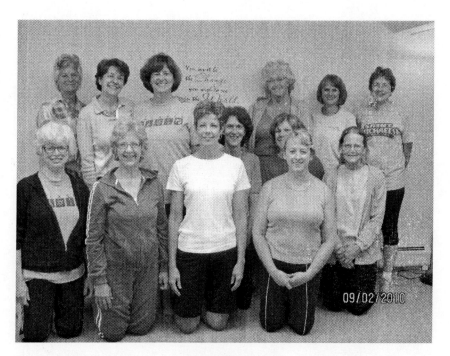

Yoga Group

Chapter 18

TRADING PAINS:
ARTHRITIS, FIBROMYALGIA AND
COMMON PAIN SYNDROMES

Once again drawing upon my encounters with people of all ages, sizes and fitness levels, it is very common to hear that the reason a person does not exercise is because of pain of one sort or another. The most common conditions associated with the pain issues are arthritis, fibromyalgia, sciatica, and back pain. While pain is a very real and difficult challenge, what is often misunderstood is that the pain is more likely to get worse with inactivity and more likely to improve with exercise. Let's start with a discussion about arthritis.

Osteoarthritis is the most common form of arthritis and probably the one that is most preventable. The number one cause of osteoarthritis is obesity. Osteoarthritis affects more women than men and generally starts to develop after the age of 40. This common condition is due to a breakdown of the cartilage within the joints which helps to cushion the end of bones to allow free movement. As the cartilage breaks down, bones rub against each other, and joint restriction occurs. Joints that were previous free flowing become stiff, movement decreases and pain results. Understandably there is then reluctance to move because of the discomfort that is felt. This then leads to a decrease in physical activity. As much as it would seem that the decrease in activities would help ease the pain, unfortunately the opposite is true. The decrease in activity leads to increased stiffness, further joint immobility and likely worsening pain.

Weight gain is both a cause and effect of arthritis. By this I mean that when a person is overweight, they are more likely to develop arthritis. Then the resulting inactivity just discussed leads to more weight gain. Take the knees for example. Our knees are made to hold up a normal weight body. As we gain weight, our joints, in this case the knees have to bear the burden of that increased weight. For every one pound of weight gained, there is a threefold increase in pressure on the knees and six times increased pressure on the hips. This excess burden causes the cartilage and joints to breakdown even more quickly eventually leading to the development of painful arthritis.

Exercise therefore is both a preventative measure and a treatment strategy for osteoarthritis. Maintaining an active lifestyle will strengthen muscles and tissues and provide more support to the joints. Joint flexibility and strength are improved with exercise as well. An added bonus is that daily activity will help you to sleep better through the night. We know that dealing with the pain of arthritis causes fatigue therefore a good night sleep indirectly improves arthritis pain by combating fatigue.

A person who already has arthritis should not feel that it is too late to start exercising. It is never too late to start being active however; there are a few key points to consider as you start. Earlier I talked about starting any exercise program slowly. For women with arthritis it is even more important to avoid over doing it. Allow joints to warm up with light exercise then increase activity as tolerated. At the end of an exercise session, icing joints can help to reduce any inflammation. If there is no contraindication; pain relievers such as acetaminophen or nonsteroidal anti-inflammatory (NSAIDs) medications taken either before or after, can help lessen the pain particularly when you are first starting your program. The Arthritis Foundation recommends acetaminophen as a first line pain relief agent. Use caution with NSAIDS especially if taking other medications as there can be interactions. Check with your health care provider or pharmacist further since they will know your personal medical history.

Another painful condition which afflicts women more often than men is fibromyalgia. This is a constellation of symptoms resulting in painful areas around the body. As earlier stated, it is quite common for people to stop exercising when they have pain from fibromyalgia. The same principles apply as discussed above relating to arthritis. The deconditioning that results will worsen the pain syndrome and the vicious cycle has started.

Some authorities say that exercise is essential for the management of fibromyalgia. There are many, many scientific studies and clinical trials evaluating different types of exercise in women with fibromyalgia which demonstrate that exercise improves overall functional ability and cardiovascular outcomes. More importantly, the degree of pain at the tenderness points has been shown to lessen in women who continue to be active. Very recently there was an analysis done looking back at nearly twenty years of literature related to fibromyalgia. The conclusion of this in-depth review was again consistent with the individual studies. The findings reinforced that exercise programs in the setting of fibromyalgia consistently improve physical function and reduced tender point pain. These effects can persist for periods of up to 2 years and in women who stay active the improvement may be even more sustained.

Another factor relating to the benefit of exercise for this chronic condition is due to the antidepressant and pain relieving effect of exercise. Earlier we discussed the release of neurohormones such as endorphins which improves ones outlook, stimulates pain relief and promotes a sense of wellbeing. The effects of endorphins can be especially beneficial in women with fibromyalgia since depression is frequently related to or a consequence of this painful syndrome. While all of these factors may lessen the discomfort associated with fibromyalgia, the added benefits of looking and feeling better can further uplift your spirit every day.

Sciatica, another fairly common painful problem as we age, is a symptom of a pinched spinal nerve as it passes from the canal into the leg. The pain can be felt as a leg cramp or much worse as a very uncomfortable sharp stabbing pain. In the case of severe pain, seeking care from a medical professional would be advised. In less significant cases, staying active may help.

When performing stress testing, it is not unusual for someone to say they don't exercise because of sciatica. The stories are of a previously active person in their forties or fifties slowing down because of pain. Admittedly certain exercises can make sciatica worse with the aggravating activity varying between individuals. At the same time, not exercising makes other things worse. I call it "trading one pain for another". The lack of exercise leads to weight gain and deconditioning. The weight gain as we age is likely to lead to arthritis as noted above or any of the other health problems discussed throughout this book. So rather than letting the sciatica get in the way, find ways to manage it and continue to exercise. Find the exercises that do not aggravate the problem as compared to others. Swimming, for example, is an excellent activity for anyone with chronic pain problems since it is an exercise that does not impose any impact on the bones and joints. Swimming also works the entire body building strength, aerobic capacity and muscle mass.

Another fabulous activity for management of many of these pain related issues is yoga. Yoga is a defined as "a physical, mental and spiritual discipline" with one of the goals being improved health. Yoga is a gentle workout that helps to work the body in a strengthening way. Yoga can be as difficult as you want it to be depending on how much you push yourself. The principles of yoga stress the importance of avoiding injury and only pushing to the limits of what you feel you are capable of without over doing it.

One of the biggest benefits of yoga is the philosophy of letting go of judging yourself or others and to do only what feels good. The yoga class I occasionally attend is comprised of women all around my age. Not only do we avoid judgment, but we get a good laugh when we hear creaking bones, can't find our balance or experience any number of age related slips. I had not participated in yoga until a few years ago and am now convinced that many of the typical aches and pains I feel related to my age such as sciatica have lessened from the yoga exercises.

The bottom line is that if you have chronic pain or even occasional pain, give exercise a try and evaluate the effects. Keeping a journal may be a great way to motivate yourself as you begin to become fitter and the pain lessens. Remember to start out very slowly. If you do too much at the beginning, you will experience soreness and it will be impossible to tell how much is your chronic pain and how much is related to working your muscles. Start now to avoid spiraling down the cycle of less activity leading to less ability and so on. Exercising can you climb the out of the spiral and up the ladder to improved health.

Chapter 19

OLDER WOMEN

Years ago, people did not focus as much on their weight and physical condition as we do now primarily because they lived in a manner that embodied healthy behaviors. Women and men who are now in their seventies, eighties and older did not routinely rely on a treadmill, elliptical, zumba class, personal trainers or any of the many other options we have available today to maintain their health. They simply stayed active, they kept moving. Some of that is obviously because of the time in which they grew up, the culture, and demands of life then compared to now. Yet, there are lessons to be learned from these older people many of whom are more fit than people much younger.

One such woman was Marguerite, a petite, vibrant, lovely lady who we all loved seeing in the office. In her early nineties, she was still traveling around the country to visit family. She did have underlying heart issues that she had to deal with but when Marguerite was diagnosed one of the first thing she asked about was exercise. Her insurance did not cover attendance at Cardiac Rehabilitation program for her heart condition so she opted to meet with a physical therapist to develop a home exercise program. Marguerite was faithful to her routine when home, and when away she was so active with her family that she could take a break from her program. She learned that staying active actually made living with her heart disease easier.

After years of living well despite her condition, Marguerite died at the age of 96 from several problems mainly related to her age. She was an inspiration to all who knew her not only because of her never-ending good nature and optimism but she also had an energy and fire difficult to match.

Another woman who comes to mind is Pauline, a 73 year old who was also undergoing a stress test for a previous episode of chest discomfort. She had osteoporosis and degeneration of several bones in her back. Pauline was within her ideal weight range and although she moved somewhat slowly, she still exercised at least three or four times a week. The activities she could do were limited from pain but Pauline said she knew activity was essential to maintain her weight and relatively good health. Even walking any distance was difficult so she swam several times a week. Pauline said that in the few weeks while she waited for her stress test she had been advised not to swim. Quickly she could feel her muscles becoming less toned and was beginning to lose her energy. Pauline was anxious to complete the stress test and rule out a heart problem so she could go back to swimming. Thankfully, her stress test was normal.

One last older woman to talk about is Mary, an 82 year old, five feet one inch tall lady who weighs 110 pounds. Throughout her life Mary has done a variety of activities although her most consistent ones were probably yoga, walking, and swimming. She was a kind of enigma in her neighborhood, walking or running long before it was popular for women to don exercise clothing and take to the streets. In her sixties, she was running enough to compete in a few foot races with one or all of her four children.

These days, Mary mostly putters around taking care of her home, watering her plants, cooking, or any number of other daily chores. One funny fact is that Mary spends about an hour taking her many vitamins and supplements since she spaces these out all the while fiddling about. The television is often on at her home mostly for her to listen to. Rarely does she sit and watch it. She still takes long strolls especially during the times she spends in New Hampshire at the beach. When moving about, it is easiest to describe her movement as a scurry rather than a walk.

Despite her age, Mary has no chronic health issues. Perhaps it is just good luck as we know there are people who are diagnosed with diseases when they have lived healthy and well. Or perhaps, Mary is an example of an older woman who has kept moving and all these years later is reaping the benefits of her healthy life style. A few years ago, Mary fell and broke her hip. Knowing that a hip fracture is very worrisome and a significant contributor to death in elderly women, this was quite a scary event. What she had going for her though was underlying good health and although her recovery was lengthy, one would never know today that she has a pin in her hip.

One very important thing that this woman did early on was instill in her then young family that being active was simply a part of life like eating, working and playing. Each night after dinner, Mary would go to the junior high school with the dog, and anyone else who would join in, for her daily walk or run. Her goal was never to be fast or to go long distances. Simply, she kept moving.

Mary is my mother and today she moves about with the ease of someone much younger than her. When I walk with my mother, I forget that she is 82 years old. But I never forget the valuable lesson she instilled in me. I learned that health is the most important asset gifted to us but one that we need to nurture rather than take for granted.

Think of an older woman who is active and still fit for her age. Undoubtly, you know a family member, friend, coworker or someone in your community like this. Think about how she has lived her life and what she does today to stay in shape. It is likely the level of activity has slowed some, but she still keeps moving. For many older individuals, it is all they know. It is a way of life. It is this way of life that this book has attempted to inspire in you. No matter what you take from this or how much you change, do something, start moving and keep moving. Stand, walk, use the stairs, avoid the drive up window. Find a friend, ask an older person if you can walk with them, be encouraged by someone around you, encourage someone you love. One cartoon I saw recently showed a patient with a doctor. The caption read: "What fits your busy schedule better, exercising one hour a day or being dead twenty four hours a day?." Although humorous, it certainly summarizes how important staying active truly is. This is the only life you have, cherish it my friends.

Additional Resources

www.nhlbi.org
http://www.nhlbi.nih.gov/health/public/heart/index.htm#chol
www.americanheart.org
www.freedieting.com/tools/calorie_calculator
http://www.nhlbi.nih.gov/health/public/heart/hbp/dash
http://www.mayoclinic.com/health/mediterranean-diet
womenfitatfifty@gmail.com
http://www.fda.gov/Food/LabelingNutrition/ConsumerInformation

Appendix A

MY EXCUSES

- Too busy
- Too tired
- Need to clean the house
- Kids need me to do something
- Too out of shape
- Exercise does not really apply to me, I don't need it
- Will look silly out there
- Don't like to exercise
- To early in the morning
- To late in the day
- Have to work late
- Too cold out
- Too hot out
- Too dark out
- Don't have the right clothes
- Don't have any clean clothes
- Don't have anyone to go with
- My favorite show is on
- Need to answer an email
- Husband wants me to stay home with him
- Not good at it
- Too damn lazy

Appendix B

REASONS TO EXERCISE

- Could benefit from losing a few pounds
- Finding it harder to move around because of the extra pounds
- Already have high blood pressure
- Need to lower cholesterol or LDL "the bad cholesterol"
- Could look and feel better if I exercised
- Would be sexier with a few less pounds
- Because my health care provider told me I should
- Favorite clothes don't fit
- Would improve my sex life
- Not sleeping as well as I should
- Am pre diabetic, diabetic or at risk of this
- Have other health related problems that might improve
- Don't have enough energy
- May inspire my partner to join me
- Need to set a better example for my kids or grandkids
- Am embarrassed by my weight gain
- Am short of breath walking up stairs
- Have a family history of heart disease, diabetes or high blood pressure
- Would feel better about myself
- Really do have enough time
- Would like to meet new people
- May help decrease pain

Appendix C

HEART DISEASE RISK FACTOR CHECKLIST

Nonmodifiable risk factors:
- Age, post menopausal
- Family History
- Man
- Race (higher risk in African Americans, Mexican Americans, American Indians, native Hawaiians and some Asian Americans)

Modifiable risk factors:
- Diabetes
- High blood pressure
- High cholesterol or high number of low density lipoprotein (LDL)
- Low number of the high density lipoprotein
- Over weight or obesity
- Inactivity
- Smoking

Appendix D

GOALS

- To feel better
- To loose _____ pounds
- To keep up with husband, friends, children, grandchildren
- To be less short of breath when doing things
- To lower blood pressure
- To cut calories eaten or to burn more calories than what is taken in
- To lower cholesterol
- To fit into some of my old clothes
- To get rid of old clothes and buy new ones in a smaller size
- To spend less money at the fast food restaurants
- To come off some medications
- To have better control of diabetes
- To avoid becoming a diabetic
- To feel better about myself
- Other:_____

Appendix E

OBJECTIVES

- Walk 3 times this week for 20 minutes each time. Do this for _____ weeks.

- After _____ weeks, walk _____ times for _____ minutes each time (increase amount)

- After _____weeks, do the same walk in _____ less minutes.

- Add _____ miles each week. (make this a small amount like ¼ mile)

- Call the local fitness center and ask about membership fees. Be sure to ask about discounts or trial incentives.

- Find one group program to join. A great place to check is your local hospital. Many have programs that may be less expensive than a fitness center.

- Try a new fitness activity that sounds fun.

- Get a buddy to work out with. Call _____ and make a date.

- Pick a day that you can work out with your friend and plan to do that for the next several weeks. _____ (day)

- Avoid eating _____(list a food) for _____ days

- Loose _____ pounds. Make this a very small number such as 1-3. If you set it too high, you will be discouraged.

- Tell at least one person what your goals and objectives are. This can help you stay motivated especially if it is a person who will check in with you as to how you are doing.

- Skip using the drive up window at the bank, coffee shop, or any other drive up every day this week. Just getting out of the car each time will help you burn calories.

- Choose a parking space half way down the lot every time you do an errand.

- Next week, choose a parking spot at the end of the lot.

- Tell your primary care provider what your health objectives are. Complete your KNOW YOUR NUMBERS chart together and work out specific goals for you.

♥♥♥♥♥ ♥♥♥♥ ♥♥♥♥♥ ♥♥♥♥♥

Appendix F
KNOW YOUR NUMBERS

LIPID PANEL
Total Cholesterol should be below 200. Lower is better to a certain point.

Triglycerides should be below 150.

LDL (bad cholesterol) goal is below 100. Lower than 70 is recommended if any known heart disease.

HDL (good cholesterol) should be higher than 40 at a minimum or 50 as a goal.

My Total Cholesterol_____
LDL_____
Triglycerides_____
HDL_____

BLOOD SUGAR

A person with no diabetes, should have a blood sugar between 70-100.

A person with diabetes should know their HbA1c (hemoglobin A1c). This should be below 7.0 or even better below 6.5.

My blood sugar_____
HbA1c _____

BLOOD PRESSURE

Normal Blood Pressure is 120/80. If you have no risk factors for cardiovascular disease, BP should be below 140/85. If you have risk factors or the presence of heart disease of diabetes, BP should be below 135/80.

My blood pressure_____

BODY MASS INDEX

Refer to the chart to determine what you BMI is and what it should be. Normal BMI is between 20-24.

My BMI _____ My target BMI is_____

♥♥♥♥♥ ♥♥♥♥ ♥♥♥♥♥ ♥♥♥♥♥

BEWARE...

WOMAN WORKING OUT.

ENTER AT YOUR OWN RISK